Organic Body Care Made Easy

147 Homemade Aromatherapy Essential Oil And Herbal Recipes For Glowing Skin And Radiant Hair

(Body Butters, Body Scrubs, Masks, Creams, Lotions, Perfumes, Bath Recipes, Massage Oils, Shampoos And More)

Samantha Stephenson

Copyright © 2014 Samantha Stephenson
All rights reserved. No part of this publication may be reproduced, distributed, or transmitted in any form or by any means, including photocopying, recording, or other electronic or mechanical methods, without the prior written permission of the publisher, except in the case of brief quotations embodied in critical reviews and certain other noncommercial uses permitted by copyright law.
ISBN-13: 978-1505435030
ISBN-10: 150543503X

DEDICATION

To Madeline, you are truly a friend indeed... and to every woman who wants to be beautiful within and without.

TABLE OF CONTENTS

INTRODUCTION	Pg 1
Why You Need To Switch To Organic Skincare	Pg 1
How Aromatherapy Works	Pg 4
Using Essential Oils Safely	Pg 8
Carrier Oils	Pg 8
Buying Essential Oils	Pg 10
Herbs For Beautiful And Healthy Skin	Pg 10
NATURAL FACE CARE	Pg 12
FACIAL CLEANSERS RECIPES	Pg 12
DIY Face Cleanser For Normal Skin	Pg 12
DIY Face Cleanser For Combination Skin	Pg 13
DIY Face Cleanser For Dry And Mature Skin	Pg 14
DIY Face Cleanser For Acne And Oily Skin	Pg 16
DIY Face Cleanser For Sensitive And Problem Skin	Pg 17
Easy Blackhead Remover	Pg 18
FACIAL SCRUBS RECIPES	Pg 19
Homemade Facial Scrub For Normal And Combination Skin	Pg 20
Homemade Facial Scrub For Dry, Mature And Damaged Skin	Pg 21
Homemade Facial Scrub For Acne And Oily Skin	Pg 22
Simple DIY Face Scrub For Combination Skin	Pg 23
FACIAL MASKS RECIPES	Pg 25
Homemade Face Mask For Normal Skin	Pg 25
Homemade Face Mask For Dry And Mature Skin	Pg 26
Homemade Face Mask For Acne And Oily Skin	Pg 27
Homemade Face Mask For Sensitive And Problem Skin	Pg 28
Orange Moisturizing Face Mask	Pg 30
Lemon Honey Mask For Acne	Pg 31
Cocoa Face Mask For Mature Skin	Pg 31

Beauty Yoghurt Mask	Pg 32
FACIAL MOISTURIZERS RECIPES	Pg 33
DIY Facial Moisturizer For Normal Skin	Pg 33
DIY Facial Moisturizer For Combination Skin	Pg 35
DIY Facial Moisturizer For Dry And Mature Skin	Pg 36
DIY Facial Moisturizer For Acne And Oily Skin	Pg 37
DIY Facial Moisturizer For Sensitive And Problem Skin	Pg 39
Tea Tree Oil Natural Face Cream	Pg 40
Homemade Vitamin C Serum	Pg 41
FACIAL STEAMS RECIPES	Pg 43
Facial Steam For Mature, Dry And Sensitive Skin	Pg 43
Facial Steam For Normal And Combination Skin	Pg 44
Facial Steam For Acne And Oily Skin	Pg 45
FACIAL SKIN TONERS RECIPES	Pg 47
DIY Facial Skin Toner For Normal And Combination Skin	Pg 47
DIY Facial Skin Toner For Mature, Dry And Sensitive Skin	Pg 48
DIY Facial Skin Toner For Acne And Oily Skin	Pg 49
NATURAL LIP CARE	Pg 50
Homemade Peppermint Lip Scrub	Pg 50
Homemade Healing Lip Balm	Pg 51
Super-Moisturizing Lip Balm	Pg 51
Cranberry Lip Gloss	Pg 52
NATURAL ORAL HYGIENE	Pg 54
Homemade Natural Toothpaste	Pg 54
Aromatherapy Germ Buster For Teeth and Gums	Pg 55
Homemade Antibacterial Mouthwash	Pg 56
Herbs And Spices Mouthwash	Pg 56
NATURAL BODY CARE	Pg 58
BODY AND BATH OILS RECIPES	Pg 58
Calming Aromatherapy Bath Oil	Pg 58
Healing Aromatherapy Bath Oil	Pg 59

Lavender Soothing Bath Oil	Pg 60
Brighter Day Aromatherapy Bath Oil	Pg 61
Soothing Aromatherapy Bath Oil	Pg 62
Sleep-Inducing Aromatherapy Bath Oil	Pg 63
BATH SALTS RECIPES	Pg 64
Luscious Lavender Bath Salts	Pg 65
Spicy And Silky Bath Salts	Pg 66
Rose-Scented Bath Salts	Pg 67
Citrus Stress Reduction Bath Salts	Pg 68
Natural Grapefruit Bath Salts	Pg 69
BUBBLE BATH RECIPES	Pg 70
Lavender Uplifting Bubble Bath	Pg 70
Sunshine Citrus Bubble Bath	Pg 71
Spicy And Silky Bubble Bath	Pg 72
Sweet Haven Bubble Bath	Pg 73
Rose Absolute Bubble Bath	Pg 74
HERBAL AROMATHERAPY BATH TEA RECIPES	Pg 76
Spicy Citrus Herbal Bath Tea	Pg 76
Oatmeal Herbal Bath Tea	Pg 78
Green Tea Herbal Bath Tea	Pg 79
MILK BATH RECIPES	Pg 81
Lavender Uplifting Milk Bath	Pg 81
Sunshine Citrus Milk Bath	Pg 82
Spicy And Silky Milk Bath	Pg 83
Sweet Haven Milk Bath	Pg 84
Rose Absolute Milk Bath	Pg 85
SHOWER STEAMER RECIPES	Pg 87
Energizing Shower Steamer	Pg 87
Anti-Stuffiness Shower Steamer	Pg 89
After Workout Shower Steamer	Pg 90
Uplifting Shower Steamer	Pg 91

Relaxing Shower Steamer	Pg 93
Spicy Shower Steamer	Pg 94
BODY BUTTER RECIPES	Pg 96
Home Spa Sensual Body Butter Massage Cream	Pg 97
Deluxe Lavender Body Butter	Pg 99
Sunshine Mango Citrus Body Butter	Pg 100
Organic Vanilla Body Cream	Pg 101
BODY SCRUB RECIPES	Pg 103
Peppermint-Citrus Salt Scrub	Pg 104
Chamomile And Oatmeal Body Scrub	Pg 105
Brown Sugar Vanilla Body Scrub	Pg 106
Yogurt And Honey Body Scrub	Pg 107
Coffee Body Scrub	Pg 108
DIY LOTION RECIPES	Pg 109
Lush Lavender DIY Body Lotion	Pg 109
Spicy Peppermint DIY Body Lotion	Pg 111
Exotic DIY Body Lotion	Pg 112
Minty Aloe DIY Sunscreen	Pg 113
DIY Bug Repellent Lotion	Pg 115
Vanilla Massage Oil Lotion Bar	Pg 116
Exotic Shea Butter Lotion Bar	Pg 117
Chocolate Peppermint Lotion Bars	Pg 118
Homemade Solid Lotion Bar	Pg 119
AROMATHERAPY MASSAGE OIL RECIPES	Pg 121
Blissful Citrus Homemade Massage Oil	Pg 121
Lavender Aromatherapy Massage Oil	Pg 122
Lavender Therapeutic Massage Oil	Pg 123
Marjoram Anti-Snoring Massage Oil	Pg 124
Stress Relief Aromatherapy Massage Oil	Pg 125
Sweet And Spicy Aphrodisiac Massage Oil	Pg 125
ESSENTIAL OILS PERFUME RECIPES	Pg 127

Mystifying Aromatherapy Perfume	Pg 127
Romantic Floral Aromatherapy Perfume	Pg 128
Energetic Aromatherapy Perfume	Pg 129
Luxurious Lavender Aromatherapy Perfume	Pg 129
Spicy And Sensual Aromatherapy Perfume	Pg 130
Sweet And Yummy Aromatherapy Perfume	Pg 131
Uplifting Aromatherapy Perfume	Pg 132
AROMATHERAPY DEODORIZING BODY POWDER RECIPES	Pg 134
Simple Deodorant Powder Recipe	Pg 134
Aromatic Lavender Dusting Powder	Pg 135
Spicy Cinnamon Dusting Powder	Pg 136
Peppermint Refreshing Dusting Powder	Pg 137
Aromatic Baby Powder	Pg 137
NATURAL HAND AND NAIL CARE	Pg 139
Anti-Aging Hand Oil	Pg 139
Aromatherapy Hand And Foot Soak For Fungus	Pg 140
Nail Whitener Soak Recipe	Pg 140
Nail Growth Soak	Pg 141
Nail Moisturizing Soak	Pg 141
NATURAL FOOT CARE	Pg 143
Spicy Salt Foot Scrub	Pg 143
Sweet And Minty Foot Scrub	Pg 144
Avocado Foot Scrub	Pg 145
Refreshing Foot Soak	Pg 146
Milky Foot Soak	Pg 147
NATURAL HAIR CARE	Pg 148
HOMEMADE SHAMPOO RECIPES	Pg 148
Dry Hair Homemade Shampoo	Pg 149
Oily Hair Homemade Shampoo	Pg 149
Thinning Hair Homemade Shampoo	Pg 150
Dandruff Homemade Shampoo	Pg 151

Blonde Hair Herbal Homemade Shampoo	Pg 152
Red Hair Herbal Homemade Shampoo	Pg 153
Dark Hair Herbal Homemade Shampoo	Pg 154
Gray Hair Herbal Homemade Shampoo	Pg 155
DIY Beer Hair Rinse	Pg 156
HOMEMADE HERBAL HAIR CONDITIONER RECIPES	Pg 157
Lavender Coconut Conditioner	Pg 158
Simple Homemade Hair Conditioner	Pg 158
Herbal Infused Vinegar Hair Rinse	Pg 159
Quick Herb And Vinegar Hair Rinse	Pg 160
NATURAL HAIR LOSS RECIPES	Pg 162
Coconut Scalp Treatment Oil	Pg 162
Hibiscus Hair Pack	Pg 163
Herbal Rinse For Hair Growth	Pg 164
Aloe Vera Scalp Massage Oil	Pg 165
Lavender And Birch Nourishing Hair Lotion	Pg 166
OTHER NATURAL HAIR CARE TREATMENT RECIPES	Pg 168
Hot Oil Conditioning Treatment	Pg 168
Honey Conditioning Hair Pack	Pg 169
Oily Hair Minty Hair Rinse	Pg 170
Dandruff Pre-Shampoo Treatment	Pg 171
Witch Hazel Dandruff Scalp Treatment	Pg 171
Homemade Nourishing Hair Treatment	Pg 172
Homemade Shealoe Butter For Hair	Pg 173
NATURAL HAIR DYE RECIPES	Pg 174
Henna Hair Coloring	Pg 174
Natural Remedy To Darken Gray Hair	Pg 174
Blonde Hair Natural Hair Dye	Pg 175
Natural Sun Streaking	Pg 176
Golden Hair Natural Hair Dye	Pg 177
Red Hair Natural Hair Dye	Pg 177

INTRODUCTION

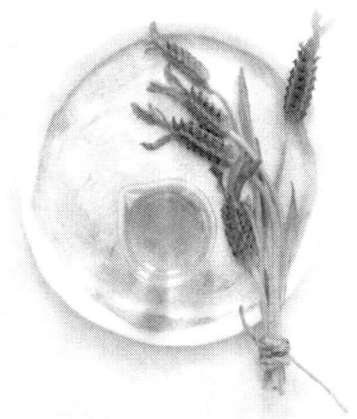

Why You Need To Switch To Organic Skincare

Many women (and men) have wondered why they have to make the switch to natural products for their skin. This is a valid query because of the thousands of skincare products on the market promising to do wonders for your skin.

Organic skincare products are better because the things you put on your skin will eventually penetrate beneath the surface into your body. The healing power of homemade natural skincare products that contain herbs or essential oils have been proven by research.

Your body understands how to work with these ingredients because they are directly from nature. On the other hand, when you apply manmade products with chemicals and synthetic addictives, your body starts to develop irritations, sensitivities and other problems.

This book is a compilation of homemade products that will enable you to enjoy the benefits of truly organic and natural skincare.

Research shows that a woman is likely to apply over 200 chemicals to her skin in the course of an ordinary day and 60% or more of these chemicals can penetrate into the bloodstream. It is therefore vital to be sure that you are using products that cannot harm you.

Using natural skincare is important if you want to safely improve the condition of your skin and maintain a fresh and youthful look. Organic ingredients are usually grown without the usage of artificial fertilizers and pesticides and the growing process is also kinder to the environment.

If you take time to read the list of ingredients on the skincare products you have been using, you will discover many chemicals with complicated long names. Several of these chemicals have negative effects on your skin and even your health. Fortunately, you have alternatives in natural products that you can make in the comfort of your own home. Here are some of the advantages of homemade organic products:

Help irritated skin

Great for sensitive skin

Does not clog pores

Anti inflammatory

No harmful ingredients

Affordable

Making Herbal And Aromatherapy Recipes Is Easy

Another advantage of making your own natural beauty products at home is that they are so easy to make. The ingredients can be bought easily and you may already have some of them in your home. They are fun, inexpensive and highly rewarding.

If you have never made natural balms, lotions and other potions before, get ready for a treat! Even if you have tried your hands on do-it-yourself beauty in the past, the 147 easy recipes in this book will simply blow your mind. Just dive in and start making body oils, lip balms, bath salts and other natural skincare stuff.

Once you start making essential oil and herbal recipes, you will never look back. Making aromatherapy goodies is a habit that you will never want to stop.

– They are easy, practical and smell truly fabulous. Now you can get rid of synthetic fragrances and never go back to them ever.

– They contain only healthy and natural ingredients that you choose by yourself.

– They possess healing powers to deal with pain, acne, stress and also kill germs.

– They help you save money.

Additionally, making aromatherapy and herbal beauty recipes is fun. You get a lot of fun when you mix, stir and smell these goodies. Your 'expertise' will increase with more practice and you will be satisfactorily rewarded with using your own aromatherapy masterpiece.

How Aromatherapy Works

Some background knowledge is important so you can have a basic understanding of the effects of essential oils on the human system. Aromatherapy has the ability to enhance your health and happiness in a variety of ways because of the properties of essential oils. The herbs that are used in some of the recipes in this book also contain valuable substances that are good for your body and health.

A Few Things To Know About Essential Oils

Essential oils are simply the distilled essences of plants. These essences are very tiny molecules that are extracted from leaves, flowers, stems and roots of flowers, herbs, shrubs, grasses and trees.

For example, if you simmer a quantity of chamomile flowers for a few minutes on the stove, you will start seeing bobs of oil forming on the surface of the water. This oil (essential oil) is the essence of the chamomile flowers. However, this description is used only as an example. The distillation/extraction processes that are used are more refined and efficient and a large quantity of the flowers will be needed to make a little oil.

The molecules of essential oils are so small that you can find as much as 40 million trillion molecules in just one drop. This very tiny size is what makes it easy for them to permeate our skin and lungs. The effect of aromatherapy is powerful because of this easy absorption.

Essential oils can be absorbed into the lungs through breathing or into the skin through massage. When they are absorbed, the molecules get into the lymphatic system and then onwards into the bloodstream. Once essential oils are in the bloodstream, they start working by fighting infection, reducing inflammation, correcting imbalances and so on.

How Aromatherapy Works Within The Body

Essential oils are full of natural chemicals which each oil having its own distinctive collection of chemicals. However, what makes these essences of plants special are substances called terpenes. Terpenes work on our bodies in various ways.

– They have the ability to boost the immune system and create an environment that is hostile to bacteria, viruses and fungi. This makes them very useful for antiseptic purposes. Lavender, Eucalyptus, Tea Tree, Lemon and Pine are examples of antiseptic oils. This is why they are used in many home cleaning products.

– They reduce inflammation. When there is inflammation in any part of your body, there will be swelling, pain and redness. Lavender, Sandalwood and Chamomile are some essential oils that have anti-inflammatory properties.

– They stimulate our cells for proper functioning and growth. For example, Rosemary, Basil and Pine can enhance the function of adrenal glands.

– They have sedative properties. Essential oils have a relaxing effect on the muscles and nervous system and this helps to alleviate tension, stress, pain, muscle cramps and spasms. Oils in this category include Geranium, Ylang Ylang, Lavender and Clary Sage.

Aromatherapy And Your Emotions

Although the main focus of this book is the effect of aromatherapy and herbal preparations on the quality of the skin, it is important to mention that essential oils also have positive effects on emotional wellbeing. When you inhale essential oils, they stimulate your olfactory nerves and signals are sent to the emotional part of your brain. This emotional part (called the limbic system), controls your breathing, blood pressure , heart rate, hormone production and memory.

When the olfactory nerves send signals to the limbic system, physiological, emotional and hormonal responses are triggered. For instance, the inhalation of Lavender essential oil triggers the brain to relax the muscles and calms the nervous system. As a result, stress is reduced and it is easier to sleep.

The stress-relieving powers of aromatherapy can be experienced in different ways. You can use various blends to calm your nerves, reduce anxiety and help your muscles to relax.

Essential Oils And Beauty

Using essential oils and herbal preparations is one of the best things you can do for your skin. You can use them to clear up acne, reduce or eliminate wrinkles, heal your body and revitalize your hair. These botanical substances have so much to offer in the area of natural skin care.

Essential oils are good for your skin because they kill bacteria, viruses and fungi thereby making your skin germ-free. They also reduce inflammation, pain and swelling that come with certain conditions and day to day stress.

Each of these essential oils is best suited to certain applications although some of them are more versatile than others. The essential oils that are used in each recipe in this book have been chosen specifically because they are the most suited for the particular purpose.

If you are just starting with essential oils, it is advisable to buy a started set that includes the following oils: Rose Geranium,

Rosemary, Thyme, Lemon, Clove, Lavender, Tea Tree, Peppermint, Chamomile and Eucalyptus.

Using Essential Oils Safely

– Do a spot test. Conduct a spot test before using any essential oil to rule out any allergic reaction. Add 1 drop of essential oil to 15 drops of a carrier oil. Rub it on a spot on your upper arm. It is safe to use if your skin shows no negative reaction after 12 hours.

– Use the appropriate dilutions of the oils before usage. Lavender is an exception to the dilution rule. It can be used neat for burns, cuts, bug bites, scrapes and so on.

– Pregnant women and individuals with conditions like hypertension, epilepsy and so on must be careful with essential oils.

– Do a spot test if you sensitive skin or allergies.

– Keep your essential oils out of reach of children.

Carrier Oils

The high potency and volatility of essential oils make it necessary to dilute them with carrier oils in bath and beauty products. Choosing the best carrier oils for your skin is easy when you have basic knowledge about their properties. The distinct quality of each carrier oil makes them more suitable for certain conditions like eczema, dryness or acne. Some are also better for specific skin types.

It is alright to experiment since trial and error will help you to discover the most appropriate carrier oil for your skin type.

Carrier Oils Quick Guide

Normal Skin: Jojoba, Apricot Kernel, Sweet Almond, Sunflower

Acne-Prone and Oily Skin: Jojoba, Grapeseed, Neem

Dry, Damaged and Aging Skin: Avocado, Sweet Almond, Calendula, Borage, Jojoba, Olive, Sea Buckthorn Kukui Nut, Rosehip,

Sensitive Skin: Avocado, Apricot Kernel, Calendula, Rice Bran, Kukui Nut, Grapeseed,

Psoriasis and Eczema Skin: Calendula, Avocado, Sweet Almond, Jojoba, Evening Primrose, Kukui Nut, Neem, Rosehip, Olive, Sea Buckthorn

Stretch Marks and Scars: Jojoba, Calendula, Rosehip, Kukui Nut, Sea Buckthorn

Bruises, Burns, Scrapes, Cuts and Stings: Rosemary, Arnica, Comfrey

Carrier Oils for Hair:

Dry or Damaged Hair: Coconut, Rosemary, Jojoba, Kukui Nut

Dandruff Hair: Jojoba, Rosemary, Neem

Hair Loss: Jojoba, Rosemary, Neem

Buying Essential Oils

Ensure that you buy essential oils from trusted and recognized aromatherapy suppliers. This field is not regulated so there are no stipulated standards. This is why quality variations are seen when you compare different merchants. Some unscrupulous suppliers also go as far as diluting the essential oils with fragrant synthetic substitutes.

Quality is very important because essential oils can penetrate your skin and mucus membranes. If the source plants are grown with pesticides, the pesticides can be carried into your cells when you use essential oils.

Herbs For Beautiful And Healthy Skin

Herbs are not just for cooking. Their power can be unlocked for the healing and protection of our bodies. The immense benefits of herbs are easily harnessed when herbs and essential oils are incorporated into homemade beauty products. Consequently Your skin will look more beautiful and radiant.

Safety Considerations For Herbal Skin Care

Herbs can help you to have clear, radiant and healthy skin but before using them in your homemade beauty products, you need to know that some of them may have negative effects on your skin. These include itching, rashes and other issues.

A simple skin test will enable you to know the herbs that are not compatible with your skin. Soak the dried herb in a little water for a while then dab the liquid on your arm. If the herb is fresh, simply squeeze it to get the juice. Wait for a day to see if your skin will develop itching, rash or redness.

Even when some herbs are used topically, they can interfere with other medicines. If you are on ongoing medication, it is vital to discuss your beauty regimen with a licensed dermatologist, a holistic herbalist or your primary health care provider.

Using Herbs For Your Skin

Herbs can be used for DIY skin care products in different ways. They can be used in facial steams, lotions, acne remedies are so on. Nevertheless, some herbs may be more suitable for your skin type than others. Notes are provided for most of the recipes in this book to make it easy to choose the most suitable for you. A basic guide is provided below:

Acne-Prone and Oily Skin: Basil, Lavender, Chamomile, Dandelion, Rosemary, Neem, Peppermint, Sage

Dry, Damaged and Aging Skin: Aloe, Clary-sage, Sage, Calendula, Borage, Comfrey, Elderflower, Marsh mallow, Peppermint

Sensitive Skin: Borage, Calendula, Lavender, Nettle, Lemon balm, Lady's mantle

NATURAL FACE CARE

FACIAL CLEANSERS RECIPES

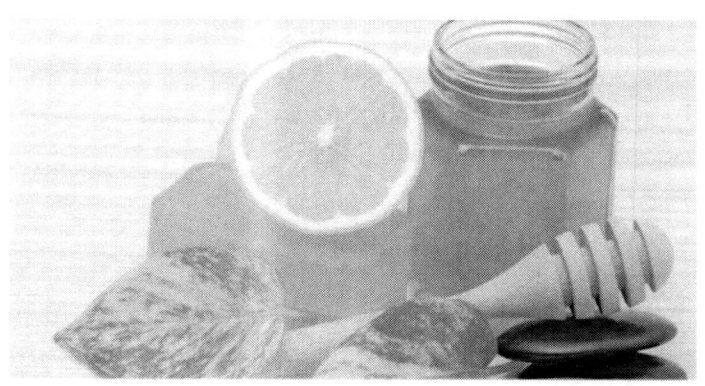

DIY Face Cleanser For Normal Skin

This effective recipe is recommended for normal skin although it is also good for other skin types.

Ingredients:

1/3 cup rose geranium hydrosol

1/3 cup lavender or rose water

1 tablespoon vegetable glycerin

1 drop sandalwood essential oil

1 drop rose geranium essential oil

8 drops lavender essential oil

1 tablespoon of pure Aloe Vera gel

Directions:

1. Combine all the ingredients in a dark glass bottle and shake.

2. Set aside to cure for at least 24 hours.

3. Dampen your face with warm water, then massage the cleanser into the skin gently.

4. Rinse your face, pat dry then moisturize.

DIY Face Cleanser For Combination Skin

This is a gentle balancing cleanser that cleanses and balances the oil production of your skin.

Ingredients:

1/2 cup rose geranium hydrosol

2 tablespoons Aloe Vera gel

2 tablespoons vegetable glycerin

3 drops petitgrain essential oil

4 drops of lavender essential oil

1 drop ylang ylang essential oil

2 drops rose geranium essential oil

Directions:

1. Combine everything in a dark glass bottle and shake well.

2. Set aside to cure for at least 24 hours.

3. Dampen your face with warm water, then massage the balancing cleanser into the skin gently.

4. Rinse your face, pat dry, apply a toner then moisturize.

DIY Face Cleanser For Dry And Mature Skin

This cleanser is terrific for mature, dry or even damaged skin. It soothes, regenerates and hydrates the cells.

Makes about 8 ounces of dry skin cleanser

Ingredients:

2 tablespoons of vegetable-based emulsifying wax

1/3 cup grapeseed or jojoba oil

2 tablespoons vegetable glycerin

1/2 teaspoon stearic acid

1 teaspoon vitamin E

1/3 cup rose geranium hydrosol

1/3 cup rose water

2 tablespoons Aloe Vera gel

10 drops grapefruit seed extract

5 drops patchouli essential oil

5 drops frankincense essential oil

5 drops palmarosa essential oil

1 drop jasmine essential oil

1 drop rose geranium essential oil

Directions:

1. Stir together emulsifying wax, oil, glycerin and stearic acid. Melt the mixture in a double boiler over low heat.

2. Remove from heat and add Vitamin E.

3. Combine the hydrosols and Aloe Vera gel in microwave-safe bowl. Microwave until lukewarm.

4. Pour the Aloe Vera gel mixture into the oil mixture, constantly stirring with a wire whisk until you have a thick and smooth combination.

5. Stir in the grapefruit seed extract and essential oils.

6. Pour the facial cleanser into an 8oz dark glass bottle. Let it cool before covering with the lid. Occasionally shake the bottle as the mixture cools so the ingredients will not separate.

7. Store in a cool and dark place.

8. Dampen your face with warm water, then massage the cleanser into the skin gently. Rinse your face, pat dry then moisturize.

DIY Face Cleanser For Acne And Oily Skin

Get rid of breakout-causing bacteria and embedded dirt with this gentle facial wash. It also soothes skin irritation and reduces redness.

Ingredients:

1/2 cup lime hydrosol

2 tablespoons Aloe Vera gel

2 tablespoons vegetable glycerin

3 drops lemongrass essential oil

3 drops petitgrain essential oil

1 drop chamomile essential oil

3 drops tea tree essential oil

5 drops grapefruit seed extract (as natural preservative)

Directions:

1. Combine all the ingredients in a dark glass bottle and shake.

2. Set aside to cure for at least 24 hours.

3. Dampen your face with warm water, then massage the cleanser into the skin gently.

4. Rinse your face, pat dry then apply a toner and moisturizer.

DIY Face Cleanser For Sensitive And Problem Skin

Easy and effective facial cleanser that washes away dirt, daily pollution and makeup. It also heals blemishes and moisturizes.

Ingredients:

Sensitive Skin:

2 drops jasmine, rose or neroli essential oil

12 drops lavender essential oil

1/2 cup of extra virgin olive oil

Psoriasis, Eczema:

15 drops patchouli essential oil

15 drops sandalwood essential oil

2 drops palmarosa essential oil

2 drops helichrysum essential oil

1 drop cedarwood or chamomile essential oil

1/2 cup of extra virgin olive oil

Directions:

1. Combine the appropriate blend above in a dark glass bottle and shake well.

2. Set aside to cure for at least 24 hours.

3. Pour a quarter-size dollop in your hand then massage into your skin. Focus on problem areas and use firm motions to work the facial cleanser deep into the pores. This will ensure the washing away of dirt, makeup, bacteria and dead skin cells.

4. Soak a clean washcloth in hot water, hold it over your face until it becomes cool then gently wipe away the facial cleanser. Rinse the cloth in hot water.

5. Repeat 2 or 3 times then finally rinse your face, pat dry, apply toner and moisturize.

The shelf life of this facial cleanser is about 3 to 6 months if stored in a cool and dark location.

Easy Blackhead Remover

Clear out pores and exfoliate your skin with the lactic acid in milk and alkalinity of baking soda.

Ingredients:

1/4 cup milk

1 tablespoon baking soda

Directions:

1. Combine the milk and baking soda. Mix well.

2. Use a soft makeup sponge to rub the mixture into blackhead-prone areas.

Rinse and repeat whenever necessary.

FACIAL SCRUBS RECIPES

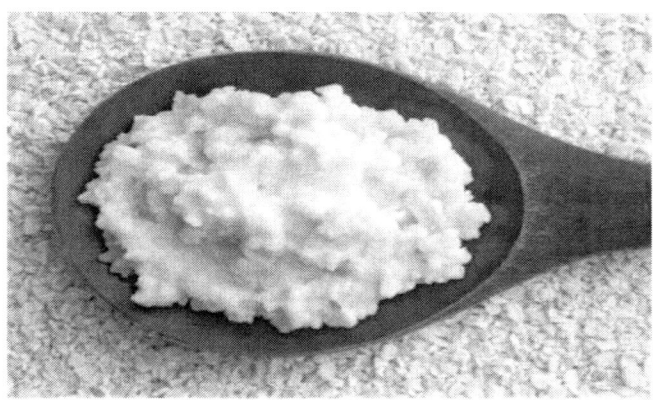

Exfoliating Your Face

Most skin experts agree that your skin should be exfoliated twice a week. But you should try to exfoliate at least once weekly. Exfoliating improves the functional ability of the dermis and also makes the skin look and feel brighter. It removes built-up makeup and residues of cosmetic products. It also enables you to get rid of dead skin cells that are clogging the surface. Your skin will be healthier and likelihood of pimple and other blemishes will decrease.

Homemade Facial Scrub For Normal And Combination Skin

This facial scrub nourishes while scrubbing away dirt, dead skin cells and bacteria.

Ingredients:

1/2 cup almonds

2 cups rolled oats

2 tablespoons of dried lavender flowers

1/2 cup powdered milk

1/2 cup cosmetic clay

4 drops of lavender essential oil

2 drops orange essential oil

2 drops frankincense essential oil

1 drop rose geranium essential oil

1 drop roman chamomile essential oil

Directions:

1. Using a clean coffee grinder and working in separate batches, grind the almonds, oats and lavender flowers. The oats and lavender flowers should be ground very fine while the almond should not be ground to powder. While grinding almonds, stop occasionally to test the texture by rubbing them between your fingers.

2. In a glass jar, combine the ground oats, almonds and lavender with milk powder and clay.

3. Add the essential oils then stir until properly combined. Store the scrub in a cool, dark place.

4. When you want to use, mix a heaping tablespoon with warm water, oil or lotion to create a paste.

5. Use gentle circular motions to massage the facial scrub into your face, avoiding the eyes and mouth.

6. Leave it on for 10 to 15 minutes. Rinse off with warm water then pat dry and apply a toner and moisturizer.

Homemade Facial Scrub For Dry, Mature And Damaged Skin

Treat your face to the rejuvenating ability of this nourishing and healing scrub. It heals imperfections and reduces wrinkles.

Ingredients:

1/2 cup almonds

2 cups rolled oats

2 tablespoons dried rose petals (optional)

1/2 cup powdered milk

2 drops patchouli essential oil

4 drops frankincense essential oil

1 drop ylang ylang essential oil

1 drop helichrysum essential oil

2 drops sandalwood essential oil

Directions:

1. Using a clean coffee grinder and working in separate batches, grind the almonds, oats and rose petals. The oats and rose petals should be ground very fine while the almond should not be ground to powder. While grinding almonds, stop occasionally to test the texture by rubbing them between your fingers.

2. In a glass jar, combine the ground oats, almonds and rose petals with milk powder.

3. Add the essential oils then stir until properly combined. Store the scrub in a cool, dark place.

4. When you want to use, mix a heaping tablespoon with warm water, oil or lotion to create a paste.

5. Use gentle circular motions to massage the facial scrub into your face, avoiding the eyes and mouth.

6. Leave it on for 10 to 15 minutes. Rinse off with warm water then pat dry and apply a toner and moisturizer.

Homemade Facial Scrub For Acne And Oily Skin

If you have acne, this is the best scrub for your face. It nourishes your skin, calms redness, absorb excess oil and cleanse away the dirt and grime.

Ingredients:

2 cups of quick cooking rolled oats

1/2 cup cosmetic clay

1/2 cup cornmeal

3 drops lavender essential oil

4 drops lemongrass essential oil

1 drop rose geranium essential oil

2 drops tea tree essential oil

Directions:

1. Using a clean coffee grinder, grind the oats to a very smooth texture.

2. In a glass jar, combine the ground oats, clay and cornmeal.

3. Add the essential oils then stir until properly combined. Store the scrub in a cool, dark place.

4. When you want to use, mix a heaping tablespoon with warm water, oil or lotion to create a paste.

5. Use gentle circular motions to massage the facial scrub into your face, avoiding the eyes and mouth.

6. Leave it on for 10 to 15 minutes. Rinse off with warm water then pat dry and apply a toner and moisturizer.

Simple DIY Face Scrub For Combination Skin

Ingredients:

1 tablespoon coffee

1 tablespoon honey

1 tablespoon baking soda

Directions:

1. Combine the ingredients in a small bowl stirring to blend thoroughly.

2. Remove all makeup, lotion, sunscreen and so on from your face. Wash your face and pat dry.

3. Apply the mixture with your fingers, massaging into your skin for about 45-60 seconds. Let it stay on for 3-5 minutes.

4. Rinse off the scrub with lukewarm water and pat dry gently.

5. Follow up with a natural facial cream or serum to lock in moisture. Repeat once weekly.

FACIAL MASKS RECIPES

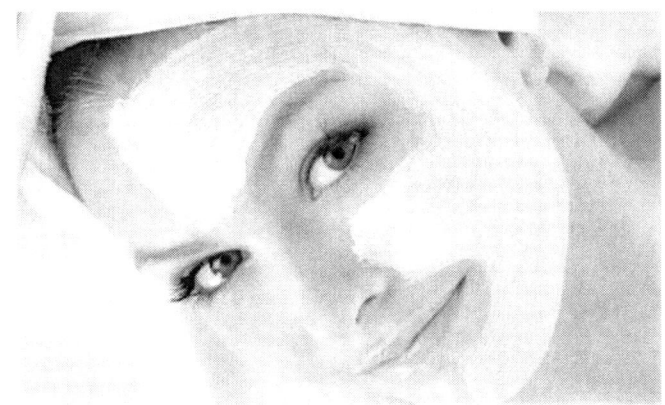

Homemade Face Mask For Normal Skin

Yummy and super-refreshing, this DIY face mask balances, hydrates and cleanses the skin. Using it weekly will help to prevent and possibly reduce the visible signs of aging.

Ingredients:

1 tablespoon cosmetic clay

1/4 teaspoon jojoba oil

1/2 teaspoon honey

1 teaspoon yogurt or milk

1 drop rose geranium essential oil

1 drop lavender essential oil

Directions:

1. In a small bowl, whisk together jojoba oil, honey, yogurt and essential oils.

2. Stir in the clay, adding a little at a time until you have a paste of desired consistency. Do not make it too thick.

3. Cleanse your face and neck area.

4. While your skin is still damp, apply the mask to your face and neck, taking care to avoid eyes and mouth. Discard any remainder.

5. Leave it on your skin for 15-20 minutes.

6. Wash off with a warm and wet washcloth then apply a toner and moisturizer.

Homemade Face Mask For Dry And Mature Skin

With easy-to-find and inexpensive items, this is a wonderful moisturizing and nourishing face mask for your skin.

Ingredients:

2 tablespoons kaolin clay

1 tablespoon sour cream or 1 egg yolk

1/2 teaspoon cider vinegar

1/2 teaspoon honey

1 teaspoon kukui nut or sweet almond oil

1 drop neroli or palmarosa essential oil

2 drops sandalwood or rose essential oil

Directions:

1. In a small bowl, whisk all the ingredients together except the kaolin clay.

2. Stir in the clay, adding a little at a time until you have a paste of desired consistency. Do not make it too thick.

3. Cleanse your face and neck area.

4. While your skin is still damp, apply the mask to your face and neck, taking care to avoid eyes and mouth. Discard any remainder.

5. Leave it on your skin for 15-20 minutes.

6. Wash off with a warm and wet washcloth then apply a toner and moisturizer.

Homemade Face Mask For Acne And Oily Skin

Simple recipe for balancing and deep cleansing acne-prone and oily skin.

Ingredients:

3 teaspoons strong herbal tea or low fat yogurt

2 teaspoons cosmetic clay

1 drop tea tree essential oil

2 drops petitgrain or lemongrass essential oil

Directions:

1. In a small bowl, combine all the ingredients. Stir in enough tea or yogurt to create a paste of desired consistency. Do not make it too thick.

2. Cleanse your face and neck area.

3. While your skin is still damp, apply the mask to your face and neck, taking care to avoid eyes and mouth. Discard any remainder.

5. Leave it on your skin for 15-20 minutes.

6. Wash off with a warm and wet washcloth then apply a toner and moisturizer.

Homemade Face Mask For Sensitive And Problem Skin

This face mask provides the soothing and healing needed by sensitive and problematic skin.

Ingredients:

Sensitive Skin Blend:

1/2 tablespoon rolled oats

1/2 teaspoon Aloe Vera juice

1/2 teaspoon evening primrose or avocado oil

1/2 teaspoon honey

1/2 tablespoon kaolin clay

1/2 teaspoon milk or yogurt

1 drop lavender essential oil

1 drop rose or jasmine essential oil

1 drop chamomile essential oil

Psoriasis & Eczema Blend:

1/2 tablespoon rolled oats

1/2 teaspoon Aloe Vera juice

1/2 teaspoon evening primrose or avocado oil

1/2 teaspoon honey

1/2 tablespoon kaolin clay

1/2 teaspoon milk or yogurt

1 drop helichrysum or chamomile essential oil

1 drop rose or jasmine essential oil

1 drop sandalwood or patchouli essential oil

Directions:

1. Using a clean coffee grinder, grind the oats to a very smooth texture.

2. Whisk together the Aloe Vera, oil and honey.

3. Stir in the oat powder and clay, adding a little at a time until you have a paste of desired consistency. Do not make it too thick.

4. Add the essential oils.

5. Cleanse your face and neck area.

6. While your skin is still damp, apply the mask to your face and neck, taking care to avoid eyes and mouth. Discard any remainder.

7. Leave it on your skin for 15-20 minutes.

8. Wash off with a warm and wet washcloth then apply a toner and moisturizer.

Orange Moisturizing Face Mask

Ingredients:

1/2 cup of instant unflavored oatmeal

Juice from 1 orange

3 tablespoons plain yogurt

2 tablespoons honey

2 teaspoons of dried orange peel

Directions:

1. In a small bowl, mix together all ingredients.

2. Stir until the mixture is well incorporated. It should be thick and not too runny. Add more oatmeal if necessary.

3. Wash and dry your face then spread the mask in an even layer, avoiding your eyes.

4. Leave on the mask for 15-30 minutes then rinse off with warm water.

Transfer any leftover to an airtight container and store in the refrigerator for up to one week or in the freezer for up to one month.

Lemon Honey Mask For Acne

The citric acid in lemon closes pores and enhances the skin's pH balance. The enzymes and nutrients in honey provide an antibacterial factor to deal with zits.

Ingredients:

1 fresh lemon

1 tablespoon organic honey

Directions:

1. Cut the lemon, squeeze the juice and remove the seeds.

2. Stir honey into the lemon juice.

3. Dampen your face and apply the mask, massaging into the skin for several minutes.

4. Rinse with lukewarm water.

Cocoa Face Mask For Mature Skin

The natural antioxidants in cocoa has and anti-aging effect on your skin.

Ingredients:

1/3 cup of natural cocoa powder (no sugar added)

2 tablespoons heavy cream

2 teaspoon cottage cheese

3 teaspoon honey

Directions:

1. Mix together everything in a large bowl.

2. Apply the mask to dampened skin then leave it on for 15-20 minutes.

3. Rinse off with warm water.

Use just once per week.

Beauty Yoghurt Mask

Greek yogurt is simply good for your face. It is high in calcium and protein as well as bacteria cultures that bring out the glow of your skin.

Ingredients:

3-5 teaspoons of Greek yogurt (vanilla or plain)

Directions:

1. Using a foundation brush or your fingers, apply a thick and even layer all over face.

2. Let the mask sit for 5-10 minutes then wash off with lukewarm water.

FACIAL MOISTURIZERS RECIPES

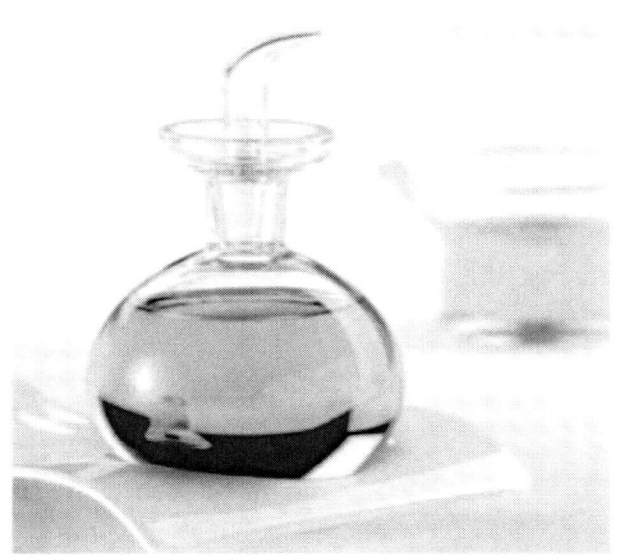

DIY Facial Moisturizer For Normal Skin

This moisturizer helps to maintain healthy hydration, enhances skin cell growth and assists in regulating the production of oil.

Ingredients:

1/3 cup apricot kernel, jojoba or kukui nut oil

2 tablespoons emulsifying wax

1 tablespoon vegetable glycerin

1/3 cup of rose geranium hydrosol

1 teaspoon vitamin E

10 drops grapefruit seed extract

1 drop palmarosa essential oil

1 drop chamomile essential oil

8 drops lavender essential oil

Directions:

1. In a double boiler on low heat, combine the oil, emulsifying wax and glycerin.

2. When everything has melted, remove from heat then add Vitamin E.

3. Warm the hydrosol in the microwave or in another pot on the stove.

4. Pour the hydrosol gently into the oil, constantly stirring with a whisk until you have a smooth and thick mixture.

5. Stir in the grapefruit seed extract and the essential oils.

6. Pour the facial moisturizer into a dark glass jar. Let it cool before covering with the lid.

7. Occasionally stir as the mixture cools so the ingredients will not separate.

8. Store in a cool and dark place. Can be stored in the refrigerator for up to 6 months.

DIY Facial Moisturizer For Combination Skin

An easy facial moisturizer recipe for protecting, hydrating and balancing the skin.

Ingredients:

1/3 cup apricot kernel or jojoba oil

2 tablespoons emulsifying wax

1 teaspoon vitamin E

1/3 cup sandalwood hydrosol

1 tablespoon Aloe Vera

10 drops grapefruit seed extract

1 drop ylang ylang essential oil

1 drop rose geranium essential oil

8 drops lavender essential oil

Directions:

1. In a double boiler on low heat, combine the oil and emulsifying wax.

2. When everything has melted, remove from heat then add Vitamin E.

3. Warm the Aloe Vera and hydrosol in the microwave or in another pot on the stove.

4. Pour the Aloe Vera/hydrosol mixture gently into the oil, constantly stirring with a whisk until you have a smooth and thick mixture.

5. Stir in the grapefruit seed extract and the essential oils.

6. Pour the facial moisturizer into a dark glass jar. Let it cool before covering with the lid.

7. Occasionally stir as the mixture cools so the ingredients will not separate.

8. Store in a cool and dark place. Can be stored in the refrigerator for up to 6 months.

DIY Facial Moisturizer For Dry And Mature Skin

Protect, nourish and revitalize mature, dry or damaged skin with this economical and effective facial moisturizer.

Ingredients:

1/3 cup apricot kernel or jojoba oil

2 tablespoons emulsifying wax

1 tablespoon vegetable glycerin

1 teaspoon vitamin E

1/3 cup rose water

10 drops grapefruit seed extract

1 drop ylang ylang essential oil

3 drops patchouli essential oil

4 drops sandalwood essential oil

1 drop rose geranium essential oil

1 drop frankincense essential oil

Directions:

1. Stir together emulsifying wax, oil and glycerin. Melt the mixture in a double boiler over low heat.

2. Remove from heat and add Vitamin E.

3. Warm the rose water in the microwave or in another pot on the stove.

4. Pour the warm rose water gently into the oil, constantly stirring with a whisk until you have a smooth and thick mixture.

5. Stir in the grapefruit seed extract and the essential oils.

6. Pour the facial moisturizer into a dark glass jar. Let it cool before covering with the lid.

7. Occasionally stir as the mixture cools so the ingredients will not separate.

8. Store in a cool and dark place. Can be stored in the refrigerator for up to 6 months.

DIY Facial Moisturizer For Acne And Oily Skin

This DIY acne cream calms and balances oily and acne-prone skin. It can also be used as a night cream.

Makes about 4 ounces

Ingredients:

1 tablespoon emulsifying wax

4 teaspoons grapeseed oil

1/2 teaspoon of stearic acid (stabilizer)

2 400-IU capsules or 1/2 teaspoon vitamin E

1 tablespoon Aloe Vera gel

1/3 cup witch hazel

5 drops grapefruit seed extract

3 drops lemon essential oil

5 drops lavender essential oil

1 drop cedarwood essential oil

1 drop rose geranium essential oil

Directions:

1. Combine the emulsifying wax, oil and stearic acid in a double boiler.

2. Let simmer, stirring occasionally until the ingredients melt together.

3. When melted, remove from heat then add Vitamin E.

4. Warm the Aloe Vera and witch hazel in the microwave or in another pot on the stove.

5. Pour the oil mixture gently into the witch hazel mixture, constantly stirring with a whisk until you have a smooth and thick mixture.

6. Stir in the grapefruit seed extract and the essential oils.

7. Pour the facial moisturizer into a dark glass jar. Let it cool before covering with the lid.

8. Occasionally stir as the mixture cools so the ingredients will not separate.

9. Store in a cool and dark place. Can be stored in the refrigerator for up to 6 months.

10. Use it each night after you have washed and toned your face.

DIY Facial Moisturizer For Sensitive And Problem Skin

This recipe is great for skin that is troubled by psoriasis, eczema, rosacea and other unpleasant skin conditions.

Ingredients:

1/3 cup calendula oil or apricot kernel oil

1 tablespoon emulsifying wax

1 tablespoon vegetable glycerin

1 teaspoon vitamin E

1/3 cup calendula hydrosol

10 drops grapefruit seed extract

1 drop chamomile essential oil

2 drops helichrysum essential oil

7 drops lavender essential oil

Directions:

1. Combine the emulsifying wax, oil and glycerin in a double boiler.

2. Let simmer, stirring occasionally until the ingredients melt together.

3. When melted, remove from heat then add Vitamin E.

4. Warm the calendula hydrosol in the microwave or in another pot on the stove.

5. Pour the warm hydrosol gently into the oil, constantly stirring with a whisk until you have a smooth and thick mixture.

6. Stir in the grapefruit seed extract and the essential oils.

7. Pour the facial moisturizer into a dark glass jar. Let it cool before covering with the lid.

8. Occasionally stir as the mixture cools so the ingredients will not separate.

9. Store in a cool and dark place. Can be stored in the refrigerator for up to 6 months.

Tea Tree Oil Natural Face Cream

This cream is good for oily as well as combo skin. It helps to clear blemishes.

Makes about 2 ounces

Ingredients:

1/2 tablespoon hazelnut oil

1 tablespoon jojoba oil

1 tablespoon rosewater

1/2 tablespoon of witch hazel extract

2 teaspoons emulsifying wax-NF

3/4 teaspoon stearic acid

40 drops tea tree essential oil

Directions:

1. Combine the hazelnut oil, jojoba oil, rosewater, witch hazel extract, emulsifying wax-NF and stearic acid in a double boiler.

2. Let simmer until the ingredients melt together.

3. Remove from the hot water then whisk for 5 minutes.

4. Add tea tree essential oil and whisk briefly then transfer to a clean glass container.

5. Continue whisking until you have a rich and thick cream. Cover the jar and refrigerate for up to 30 days.

Homemade Vitamin C Serum

This serum lightens hormonal pigmentation, tightens the skin and reduces the occurrence of wrinkles. Rub it on every night before going to bed and you will see great results within a few short weeks.

Ingredients:

1 teaspoon of Vitamin C powder

2 teaspoon of vegetable glycerin

Directions:

1. Mix the ingredients in a small bowl.

2. Crush the crystals until totally dissolved (you can add a very small bit of distilled water to make it easier).

3. Pour the serum carefully into a dark colored glass bottle.

4. Cleanse your face and neck then apply 3-4 drops of the serum and massage gently until fully absorbed. Use every night.

Note - You may experience temporary redness but that is normal with Vitamin C serum. However, if there is burning sensation, wash off with cool water then reduce the amount of Vitamin C powder in the recipe.

FACIAL STEAMS RECIPES

Facial Saunas

Aromatherapy herbal facial steams provide an excellent way to have facial saunas in your home once a week to cleanse and also revitalize your skin. They are especially good for acne-prone and oily skin. When you use face steams, pores open up and your skin is able to easily get rid of deep-down dirt, grime and excess oil. You can also have a facial sauna before using a facial mask.

Facial Steam For Mature, Dry And Sensitive Skin

The combination of ingredients in this recipe creates a steam that soothes dry or irritated skin.

Ingredients:

2 tablespoons dried elder flower

2 tablespoons dried rose petals

2 tablespoons dried chamomile

1 drop chamomile essential oil

2 drops helichrysum essential oil

5 drops frankincense essential oil

1 drop rose essential oil

2 drops sandalwood essential oil

Directions:

1. Combine the flowers and dried herbs in a dark glass jar.

2. Drop in each of the essential oils and shake well.

3. Set aside to cure for at least 24 hours.

4. Usage: Throw a handful of the mixture in a large pot, add 1-2 quarts of water then bring to a boil.

5. Remove from heat and let steep, covered for about 5 minutes.

6. Remove the lid, place the pot on a low table then using a towel, make a tent on your head together with the pot of steaming herbs.

7. Stay in this tent for about 10 minutes. Come out for air as necessary. Do let your face burn.

Facial Steam For Normal And Combination Skin

The sweetly scented steam will cleanse, open up and soothe your skin.

Ingredients:

2 tablespoons dried rose petals

2 tablespoons dried chamomile

2 tablespoons of dried lavender flowers

2 tablespoons dried calendula

2 drops palmarosa essential oil

5 drops lavender essential oil

1 drop chamomile essential oil

1 drop ylang ylang essential oil

1 drop rose geranium essential oil

Directions:

1. Combine the flowers and dried herbs in a dark glass jar.

2. Drop in each of the essential oils and shake well.

3. Set aside to cure for at least 24 hours.

4. Usage: Throw a handful of the mixture in a large pot, add 1-2 quarts of water then bring to a boil.

5. Remove from heat and let steep, covered for about 5 minutes.

6. Remove the lid, place the pot on a low table then using a towel, make a tent on your head together with the pot of steaming herbs.

7. Stay in this tent for about 10 minutes. Come out for air as necessary. Do let your face burn.

Facial Steam For Acne And Oily Skin

The cleaning, healing and refreshing provided by this face steam are vital for oily and acne-prone skin.

Ingredients:

1/4 cup dried parsley leaves

1/4 cup dried rosemary leaves

2 tablespoons dried peppermint leaves

1/4 cup dried lavender flowers

5 drops lemon or bergamot essential oil

10 drops lavender essential oil

Directions:

1. Combine the flowers and dried herbs in a dark glass jar.

2. Drop in each of the essential oils and shake well.

3. Set aside to cure for at least 24 hours.

4. Usage: Throw a handful of the mixture in a large pot, add 1-2 quarts of water then bring to a boil.

5. Remove from heat and let steep, covered for about 5 minutes.

6. Remove the lid, place the pot on a low table then using a towel, make a tent on your head together with the pot of steaming herbs.

7. Stay in this tent for about 10 minutes. Come out for air as necessary. Do let your face burn.

FACIAL SKIN TONERS RECIPES

Why Facial Skin Toners Are Necessary

Incorporating the use of a face toner in your skincare routine is vital if you want to see an improvement in the overall appearance of your skin. It also helps to balance the production of oil. A facial toner also provides a quick way to give your face its nightly beauty treatment whenever you cannot make the effort for cleansing your face properly before bed. All you have to so is to spritz it on, wipe it off and apply a moisturizer.

DIY Facial Skin Toner For Normal And Combination Skin

Ingredients:

1 cup of rose geranium hydrosol

1 drop palmarosa essential oil

1 drop rose geranium essential oil

1 drop ylang ylang essential oil

1 drop patchouli essential oil

7 drops lavender essential oil

Directions:

1. Mix the ingredients together in a dark glass bottle. Shake well.

2. Set aside to cure for at least 24 hours.

3. Usage: Shake the bottle, saturate a cotton pad with the toner and wipe it gently over your face and neck area. Avoid your eyes.

4. Follow with a facial oil or moisturizer.

DIY Facial Skin Toner For Mature, Dry And Sensitive Skin

This is a gentle anti-aging facial toner that reduces wrinkles, soothes skin irritation and promotes healthy skin.

Ingredients:

1 cup of rose hydrosol

1 teaspoon of vegetable glycerin (optional)

3 drops sandalwood essential oil

3 drops frankincense essential oil

3 drops lavender essential oil

1 drop chamomile essential oil

Directions:

1. Mix the ingredients together in a dark glass bottle. Shake well.

2. Set aside to cure for at least 24 hours.

3. Usage: Shake the bottle, saturate a cotton pad with the toner and wipe it gently over your face and neck area. Avoid your eyes.

4. Follow with a facial oil or moisturizer.

DIY Facial Skin Toner For Acne And Oily Skin

This toner removes excess oil, tightens pores and kills bacteria that cause acne.

Ingredients:

1 cup witch hazel

3 drops petitgrain essential oil

3 drops palmarosa essential oil

3 drops tea tree essential oil

3 drops lemongrass essential oil

1 drop rose geranium essential oil

Directions:

1. Mix the ingredients together in a dark glass bottle. Shake well.

2. Set aside to cure for at least 24 hours.

3. Usage: Shake the bottle, saturate a cotton pad with the toner and wipe it gently over your face and neck area. Avoid your eyes.

4. Follow with a facial oil or moisturizer.

NATURAL LIP CARE

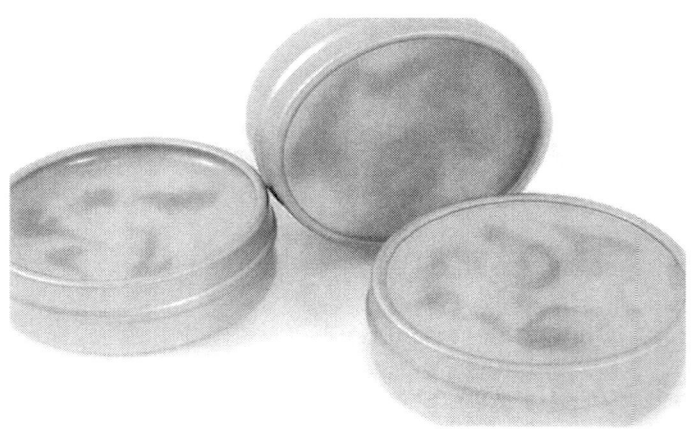

Homemade Peppermint Lip Scrub

The results of this recipe are simply amazing. The peppermint feels refreshing especially early in the morning.

Ingredients:

2 tablespoons olive oil

1 teaspoon granulated sugar

A few drops of peppermint extract

Directions:

1. Simply mix together the ingredients in a small bowl.

2. Transfer the mixture into a jar.

Homemade Healing Lip Balm

This lip balm seals in moisture by sinking into your lips to create an effective barrier. Use it with a lip scrub to remove dead, dry and scaly skin.

Ingredients:

1 tablespoon of grated beeswax

1 dash of organic raw honey

1 tablespoon virgin coconut oil

2 vitamin E capsules

20 drops tea tree or peppermint essential oil (optional)

Directions:

1. Melt the beeswax in a double boiler. When beeswax starts to melt, add the honey and coconut oil and melt together.

2. Remove from the heat then add vitamin E, stirring with a metal spoon to combine.

3. Let cool for a while, stir in the essential oil then pour into a tube or container and let cool completely.

4. Apply when needed.

Super-Moisturizing Lip Balm

Pamper and protect your lips with this balm when the weather turns dry.

Ingredients:

1 teaspoon organic raw Shea butter

2 teaspoons beeswax pastilles

3 teaspoons organic unrefined coconut oil

10 drops peppermint essential oil

10 drops tangerine essential oil

Directions:

1. In a small saucepan, combine the Shea butter, beeswax and coconut oil then melt on low heat.

2. Remove from the heat then add the essential oils, stirring to combine.

3. Using a funnel, pour the liquid into lip balm tubes. Set aside to cool.

Cranberry Lip Gloss

Beautiful, moisturizing and glistening lip balm made simply from four natural ingredients.

Ingredients:

12 fresh cranberries

1 teaspoon honey

1 tablespoon of avocado oil (or any vegetable oil)

1 capsule Vitamin E (or 2 drops)

Directions:

1. Combine cranberries, honey, avocado oil and Vitamin E in a saucepan and bring to a boil on the stovetop.

2. Use a wooden spoon to crush the cranberries until you have enough color.

3. Let the mixture cool for 10 minutes then strain it through cheese cloth to remove the cranberry bits.

4. Let cool completely then spoon into a lip balm tube.

NATURAL ORAL HYGIENE

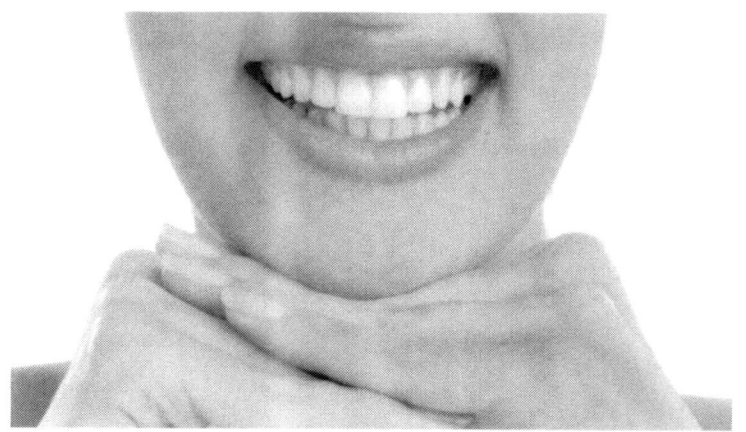

Homemade Natural Toothpaste

Ingredients:

3 tablespoons coconut oil

3 tablespoons baking soda

25 drops of peppermint essential oil

1 packet stevia

2 teaspoon vegetable glycerin

Directions:

1. Mash the baking soda and coconut oil together in a jar.

2. Mix in the other ingredients to create a paste.

3. Store with the lid covered tightly. Dip in your toothbrush whenever you want to use.

Aromatherapy Germ Buster For Teeth and Gums

Ingredients:

1 teaspoon peppermint essential oil

1/2 teaspoon spearmint essential oil

1/2 teaspoon cinnamon essential oil

1/2 teaspoon clove essential oil

1/2 teaspoon tea tree essential oil

1/2 teaspoon lemon essential oil

4 tablespoons of a carrier oil

Directions:

1. Blend the ingredients together in a bottle.

2. After brushing your teeth, add 2 drops to your toothbrush then brush your teeth and gum gently.

3. Rinse with water and spit it out. Do not swallow.

Homemade Antibacterial Mouthwash

The antifungal and antibacterial properties will help you to keep bad breath away.

Ingredients:

½ cup of distilled water

2 tablespoons baking soda

2 drops peppermint essential oil

2 drops tea tree essential oil

Directions:

1. Mix everything together in a mason jar.

2. Shake before each use.

3. Usage: Swish 2 or 3 teaspoons of the mixture in your mouth for about 1 minute. Do not swallow.

Herbs And Spices Mouthwash

Improve gum health with this herbal mouthwash.

Ingredients:

8 ounces of vodka

1 teaspoon clove powder

2 tablespoons of dried peppermint leaf

2 tablespoons of dried plantain leaf

1 tablespoon rosemary leaf

20 drops of peppermint or cinnamon essential oil

Directions:

1. In a pint size mason jar, combine the herbs.

2. Pour boiling water on the herbs to dampen them.

3. Add the vodka to the jar.

4. Cover the jar tightly and place it in a cool and dark place for 2 or 3 weeks. Shake it at least once a day.

5. After 2 to 3 weeks, strain with a very fine mesh or cheesecloth. Keep the liquid and discard the herbs.

6. Transfer the liquid into a glass jar. Add the essential oils, cover with lid and shake.

7. Usage: Mix 40 drops of the tincture with 2 teaspoon of water and swish for about 1 minute in your mouth.

NATURAL BODY CARE

BODY AND BATH OILS RECIPES

Soothe Your Nerves And Smoothen Your Skin With Bath And Body Preparations

A scented warm bath gives your body the opportunity to recover from the wear and tear of the day. These homemade bath recipes will help to work out the kinks to relax and get rid of stress. The essential oils nourish your body at deeper levels while the carrier oils provide hydration and nourishment for your skin.

Calming Aromatherapy Bath Oil

This bath recipe balances your nerves, de-stresses and helps with PMS.

Ingredients:

36 drops lavender essential oil

2 drops clary sage essential oil

2 drops chamomile essential oil

2 drops cypress essential oil

2 drops rose geranium essential oil

4 ounces jojoba or sweet almond oil (or other carrier oil of your choice)

Directions:

1. Mix together all ingredients in a dark glass bottle.

2. Store in a cool and dark place.

3. Usage: Pour about 1 tablespoon into warm bath water and swirl it around to disperse.

4. Slide into the water and relax for 20 to 30 minutes.

Healing Aromatherapy Bath Oil

This aromatherapy bath oil contains eucalyptus and other oils that decongest stuffiness, energize sore bodies, boost energy and improve your concentration.

Ingredients:

15 drops eucalyptus essential oil

10 drops sweet orange essential oil

10 drops peppermint essential oil

5 drops tea tree essential oil

5 drops rosemary essential oil

4 ounces jojoba, apricot kernel oil (or other carrier oil of your choice)

Directions:

1. Mix together all ingredients in a dark glass bottle.

2. Store in a cool and dark place.

3. Usage: Pour about 1 tablespoon into warm bath water and swirl it around to disperse.

4. Slide into the water and relax for 20 to 30 minutes.

5. You could also use this blend to reduce coughing and congestion by rubbing it directly on your chest and back.

Caution: Do not use prior to sun exposure because the orange essential oil may cause sunburn. Do not use if you are epileptic or have high blood pressure because of the rosemary and eucalyptus oils.

Lavender Soothing Bath Oil

Unwind in the bath with this pain-relieving, relaxing and sleep-inducing blend. It is good for insomnia, stress, colds and flu.

Ingredients:

10 drops lavender essential oil

1 drop cedarwood essential oil

5 drops marjoram essential oil

5 drops frankincense essential oil

4 ounces jojoba or sweet almond oil (or other carrier oil of your choice)

Directions:

1. Mix together all ingredients in a dark glass bottle.

2. Store in a cool and dark place.

3. Usage: Pour about 1 tablespoon into warm bath water and swirl it around to disperse.

4. Slide into the water and relax for 20 to 30 minutes.

Brighter Day Aromatherapy Bath Oil

The sweet citrus scent of this blend has a mood-lifting power that will lighten you up and get rid of misery, crankiness and tiredness. Great for depression, menopause and PMS.

Ingredients:

10 drops sweet orange essential oil

10 drops bergamot essential oil

5 drops rose geranium essential oil

4 ounces grapeseed oil or jojoba (or other carrier oil of your choice)

Directions:

1. Mix together all ingredients in a dark glass bottle.

2. Store in a cool and dark place.

3. Usage: Pour about 1 tablespoon into warm bath water and swirl it around to disperse.

4. Slide into the water and relax for 20 to 30 minutes.

Caution: Do not use prior to sun exposure because the citrus essential oils may cause sunburn.

Soothing Aromatherapy Bath Oil

This yummy bath blend has a deep woodsy scent that is good for men. Within a few minutes in a warm bath, you will feel your stress melting away. The bath oil also revitalizes dry or aging skin and is good for skin issues like psoriasis and eczema.

Ingredients:

30 drops of sandalwood essential oil

2 drops cedarwood essential oil

12 drops lavender essential oil

4 ounces jojoba or sweet almond oil (or other carrier oil of your choice)

Directions:

1. Mix together all ingredients in a dark glass bottle.

2. Store in a cool and dark place.

3. Usage: Pour about 1 tablespoon into warm bath water and swirl it around to disperse.

4. Slide into the water and relax for 20 to 30 minutes.

Sleep-Inducing Aromatherapy Bath Oil

A rich and sensuous blend that calms your nerves, help your muscles relax and makes your mind quite so you can easily fall into a peaceful sleep. It is also good for healing damaged skin and wrinkles reduction.

Ingredients:

16 drops orange essential oil

20 drops of lavender essential oil

4 drops clary sage essential oil

1 drop ylang ylang

1 drop vetiver essential oil

4 ounces of carrier oil of your choice

Directions:

1. Mix together all ingredients in a dark glass bottle.

2. Store in a cool and dark place.

3. Usage: Pour about 1 tablespoon into warm bath water and swirl it around to disperse.

4. Slide into the water and relax for 20 to 30 minutes.

Caution: Do not use prior to sun exposure because the orange essential oil may cause sunburn.

BATH SALTS RECIPES

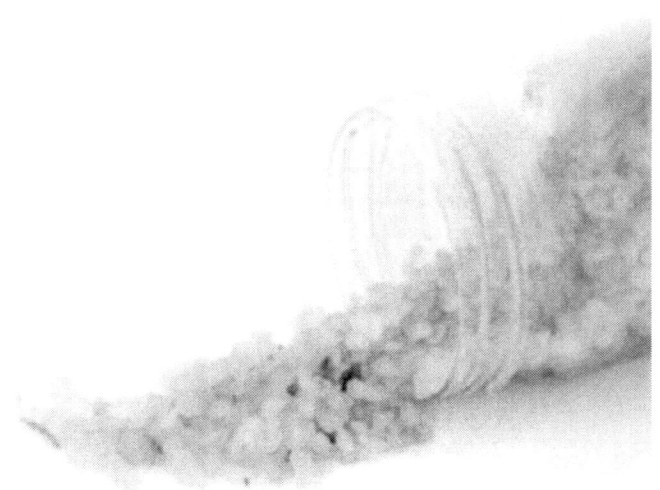

Pretty, Fragrant And Powerful

Bath salts are so easy to make, you will wonder why you never made them before. Make favorite scents for yourself and a batch for friends and loved ones! Bath salts cleanse, heal, detoxify and relieve pain. Pain is relieved when tight muscles are relaxed and inflammation is reduced. In addition, your nerves will be soothed, stress will be brought down and your body will be recharged. Overall, you will get a nice boost of energy each time you use bath salts.

Luscious Lavender Bath Salts

When you are tired and moody, cheer yourself up with the bubbles of this soothing, comforting and warming bubble bath salt. Good for muscle spasm, arthritis pain and general body discomfort.

Makes about 3 cups

Ingredients:

3 cups dead sea salt

1 tablespoon vegetable glycerin

1/4 cup liquid castile soap

1 teaspoon white sugar

2 drops rose geranium essential oil

12 drops lavender essential oil

1 drop chamomile essential oil

1 drop clary sage essential oil

8 drops blue and 2 drops red food coloring (optional)

Directions:

1. Scoop the salt into a glass, ceramic or metal bowl.

2. In another bowl, combine the remaining ingredients and use a metal spoon to stir together thoroughly.

3. Stir the soap mixture into the salt until well mixed.

4. Transfer the bath salts into a clean dark glass jar. Set aside to cure for at least 24 hours.

5. Usage: 1 cup of the bath salt per bath. Pour it into warm bath water and swirl it around to disperse.

6. Slide into the water and relax for 20 to 30 minutes.

Spicy And Silky Bath Salts

Sensual, delicious and exotic, this aphrodisiac bath salts will lift your mood, soothe your nerves and loosen your muscles. Its earthy scent also makes it ideal for men.

Makes about 3 cups

Ingredients:

2 cups of Epsom salt

1 cup of dead sea salt

1/2 cup of baking soda

3 drops frankincense essential oil

10 drops sandalwood essential oil

1 drop ceradwood essential oil

2 drops patchouli essential oil

6 drops red and 4 drops yellow food coloring (optional)

Directions:

1. In a glass, ceramic or metal bowl, combine salts and baking soda then stir together with a metal spoon.

2. Add essential oils and the food coloring (if using). Stir to mix thoroughly.

3. Transfer the bath salts into a clean dark glass jar. Set aside to cure for at least 24 hours.

4. Usage: 1 cup of the bath salt per bath. Pour it into warm bath water and swirl it around to disperse.

5. Slide into the water and relax for 20 to 30 minutes.

Caution: Individuals with high blood pressure should replace Epsom salt with sea salt.

Rose-Scented Bath Salts

Use this bath salts when you want to feel calm, relaxed and happy. Good for daily stress, depression, grief, menopause and PMS.

Ingredients:

3 cups dead sea salt or Himalayan salt

1/2 cup of baking soda

4 drops rose essential oil

6 drops palmarosa essential oil

1 drop ylang ylang essential oil

2 drops patchouli essential oil

4 drops rose geranium essential oil

10 drops of red food coloring (optional)

Directions:

1. In a glass, ceramic or metal bowl, combine salt and baking soda then stir together with a metal spoon.

2. Add essential oils and the food coloring (if using). Stir to mix thoroughly.

3. Transfer the bath salts into a clean dark glass jar. Set aside to cure for at least 24 hours.

4. Usage: 1 cup of the bath salt per bath. Pour it into warm bath water and swirl it around to disperse.

5. Slide into the water and relax for 20 to 30 minutes.

Citrus Stress Reduction Bath Salts

Stress and tension melt away as you soak in warm bath water with this uplifting bath salts that calms and balances your nerves. It is also good for acne-prone and oily skin because it cleanses the skin, heals blemishes and reduces oil production.

Ingredients:

2 cups of dead sea salt or Epsom salt

1 cup of sea salt

1/2 cup of baking soda

3 drops lavender essential oil

6 drops sweet orange essential oil

6 drops bergamot essential oil

4 drops red and 4 drops of yellow food coloring (optional)

Directions:

1. In a glass, ceramic or metal bowl, combine salts and baking soda then stir together with a metal spoon.

2. Add essential oils and the food coloring (if using). Stir to mix thoroughly.

3. Transfer the bath salts into a clean dark glass jar. Set aside to cure for at least 24 hours.

4. Usage: 1 cup of the bath salt per bath. Pour it into warm bath water and swirl it around to disperse.

5. Slide into the water and relax for 20 to 30 minutes.

Caution: Do not use prior to sun exposure because sweet orange and bergamot may cause sunburn.

Natural Grapefruit Bath Salts

Ingredients:

1 toe of a nylon stocking or cheesecloth

1 cup sea salt

2 drops pink food coloring

4 drops essential oil (choose your favorite fragrance)

Directions:

1. Place the salt on the cheesecloth or in the toe of the stocking.

2. Add the food coloring and essential oil. Fold up the cheesecloth or toe of stocking and tie with a string.

3. Add the bag to your bath water and let it disperse slowly into the water. Soak for 20-30 minutes.

BUBBLE BATH RECIPES

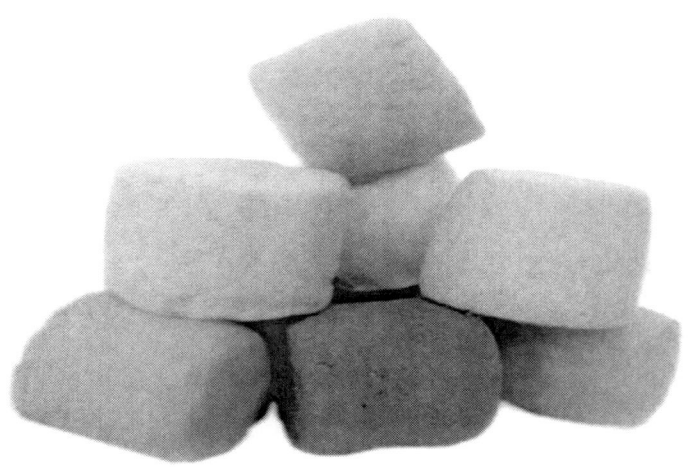

Have Fun With Bubble Bath Products

Use any of the recipes below whenever you want to have fun in the tub. They provide a nice way to try a variety of scents without spending much money.

Lavender Uplifting Bubble Bath

Ingredients:

1 1/2 cups of liquid castile soap

1/2 tablespoon white sugar

2 tablespoons vegetable glycerin

5 drops lavender essential oil

4 drops lemon essential oil

1 drop chamomile essential oil

5 drops of your preferred food coloring

Directions:

1. In a large ceramic or glass bowl, stir together all the ingredients gently.

2. Transfer the bubble bath into a clean dark glass jar. Set aside to cure for at least 24 hours. Store in a cool and dark place.

3. Usage: 1/4 cup of the bubble bath per bath. Pour it into warm bath water and swirl it around to disperse.

4. Slide into the water and relax for 20 to 30 minutes.

Sunshine Citrus Bubble Bath

Ingredients:

1 1/2 cups of liquid castile soap

1/2 tablespoon white sugar

2 tablespoons vegetable glycerin

5 drops bergamot essential oil

4 drops orange essential oil

1 drop ylang ylang or rose geranium essential oil

5 drops of your preferred food coloring

Directions:

1. In a large ceramic or glass bowl, stir together all the ingredients gently.

2. Transfer the bubble bath into a clean dark glass jar. Set aside to cure for at least 24 hours. Store in a cool and dark place.

3. Usage: 1/4 cup of the bubble bath per bath. Pour it into warm bath water and swirl it around to disperse.

4. Slide into the water and relax for 20 to 30 minutes.

Caution: Do not use prior to sun exposure because orange and bergamot may cause sunburn.

Spicy And Silky Bubble Bath

Ingredients:

1 1/2 cups of liquid castile soap

1/2 tablespoon white sugar

2 tablespoons vegetable glycerin

5 drops lavender essential oil

4 drops sandalwood essential oil

1 drop clove essential oil

5 drops of your preferred food coloring

Directions:

1. In a large ceramic or glass bowl, stir together all the ingredients gently.

2. Transfer the bubble bath into a clean dark glass jar. Set aside to cure for at least 24 hours. Store in a cool and dark place.

3. Usage: 1/4 cup of the bubble bath per bath. Pour it into warm bath water and swirl it around to disperse.

4. Slide into the water and relax for 20 to 30 minutes.

Caution: Leave out clove if you have sensitive skin.

Sweet Haven Bubble Bath

Ingredients:

1 1/2 cups of liquid castile soap

1/2 tablespoon white sugar

2 tablespoons vegetable glycerin

6 drops vanilla absolute essential oil

5 drops of your preferred food coloring

Directions:

1. In a large ceramic or glass bowl, stir together all the ingredients gently.

2. Transfer the bubble bath into a clean dark glass jar. Set aside to cure for at least 24 hours. Store in a cool and dark place.

3. Usage: 1/4 cup of the bubble bath per bath. Pour it into warm bath water and swirl it around to disperse.

4. Slide into the water and relax for 20 to 30 minutes.

Rose Absolute Bubble Bath

Ingredients:

1 1/2 cups of liquid castile soap

1/2 tablespoon white sugar

2 tablespoons vegetable glycerin

3 drops rose absolute essential oil

2 drops palmarosa essential oil

1 drop rose geranium essential oil

5 drops of your preferred food coloring

Directions:

1. In a large ceramic or glass bowl, stir together all the ingredients gently.

2. Transfer the bubble bath into a clean dark glass jar. Set aside to cure for at least 24 hours. Store in a cool and dark place.

3. Usage: 1/4 cup of the bubble bath per bath. Pour it into warm bath water and swirl it around to disperse.

4. Slide into the water and relax for 20 to 30 minutes.

HERBAL AROMATHERAPY BATH TEA RECIPES

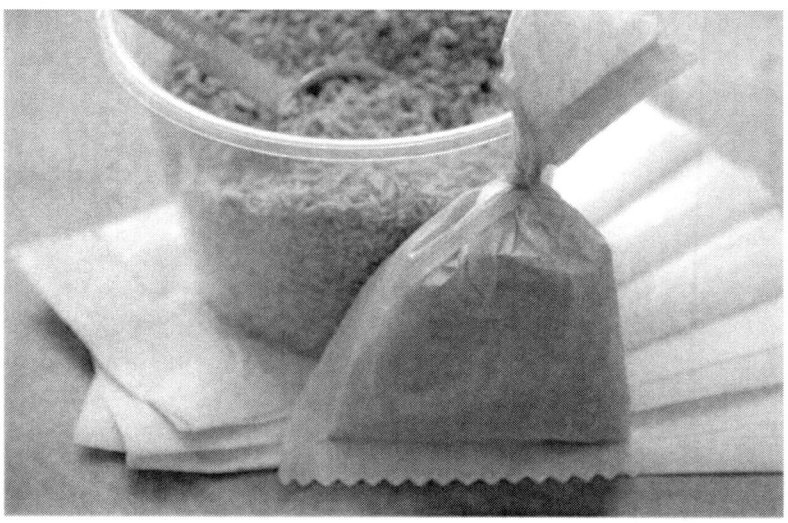

Heal Your Body... Heal Your Soul

Herbal aromatherapy bath tea recipes are effective when you want to give your body some tender loving care. The fragrance and healing ability of essential oils blend perfectly with herbs to nourish your skin, calm nerves, relax your muscles and elevate your mood.

Spicy Citrus Herbal Bath Tea

Get ready to be enchanted by the sweet, rich and spicy scent of this aromatherapy bath recipe. Excellent for easing muscle and joint pain and relaxing your body.

Ingredients:

1/2 cup lavender flowers

1/2 cup dried lemongrass

2 tablespoons of chopped licorice root (optional)

2 tablespoons whole cloves

3 drops palmarosa essential oil

3 drops lavender essential oil

3 drops lemongrass essential oil

Directions:

1. In a dark glass jar, combine lavender flowers, lemongrass and licorice root.

2. Place the cloves in a plastic bag and hit with a hammer to break them into smaller pieces and release the scent. Add cloves to the glass jar.

3. Add the essential oils and stir everything together gently with a metal spoon.

4. Cover the jar and set it aside to cure for at least 24 hours.

5. Usage: Put a few spoonfuls in a small muslin or organza drawstring bag. You may also use cheesecloth and tie with a string.

6. Bring water to a boil in a kettle then steep the herbal bath tea bag for about 10 minutes.

7. Pour the herbal tea water into your bath water then throw in the bag.

8. Slide into the water and relax for 20 to 30 minutes.

8. Do not rinse your body. Just pat dry with a towel then apply a natural body lotion.

Oatmeal Herbal Bath Tea

This nourishing oatmeal bath recipe soothes and moisturizes dry and problematic skin. It also relieves irritation, itchiness and inflammation. Good for psoriasis, eczema and acne.

Ingredients:

2 cups of rolled oats

3 tablespoons chamomile flowers

3 tablespoons lavender flowers

3 drops palmarosa essential oil

4 drops of lavender essential oil

4 drops chamomile essential oil

Directions:

1. Grind the oats in your blender until you have a coarse powder.

2. In a large bowl, combine the ground oats with lavender and chamomile flowers.

3. Add the essential oils and stir everything together gently with a metal spoon. Combine everything in a dark glass jar.

4. Cover the jar and set it aside to cure for at least 24 hours.

5. Usage: Put a few spoonfuls in a small muslin or organza drawstring bag. You may also use cheesecloth and tie with a string.

6. Bring water to a boil in a kettle then steep the herbal bath tea bag for about 10 minutes.

7. Pour the herbal tea water into your bath water then throw in the bag.

8. Slide into the water and relax for 20 to 30 minutes.

8. Do not rinse your body. Just pat dry with a towel then apply a natural body lotion.

Green Tea Herbal Bath Tea

Gentle and nourishing herbal bath tea that soothes nerves and softens the skin.

Ingredients:

1/2 cup lavender flowers

1/2 cup rose petals

1/4 cup green tea leaves (such as jasmine or rose flavored tea)

1 drop rose geranium essential oil

3 drops lavender essential oil

3 drops rose or palmarosa essential oil

Directions:

1. In a dark glass jar, combine the lavender flowers, rose petals and tea leaves.

2. Add the essential oils and stir everything together gently with a metal spoon.

4. Cover the jar and set it aside to cure for at least 24 hours.

5. Usage: Put a few spoonfuls in a small muslin or organza drawstring bag. You may also use cheesecloth and tie with a string.

6. Bring water to a boil in a kettle then steep the herbal bath tea bag for about 10 minutes.

7. Pour the herbal tea water into your bath water then throw in the bag.

8. Slide into the water and relax for 20 to 30 minutes.

8. Do not rinse your body. Just pat dry with a towel then apply a natural body lotion.

MILK BATH RECIPES

Yummy And Super-Easy

Milk bath recipes are good for people who want to rejuvenate the vitality of their skin. When your skin is feeling dry, soak for a few minutes in one of the healing and soothing preparations below. Milk softens the skin and removes the layer of dead cells that are clogging the surface. Use milk with higher fat content to get more nourishment. The essential oils in each recipe also provide additional benefits.

Lavender Uplifting Milk Bath

Ingredients:

2 cups of whole powdered milk

1/4 cup baking soda

1/2 cup cornstarch

10 drops lavender essential oil

9 drops lemon essential oil

1 drop chamomile essential oil

Directions:

1. In a dark glass jar, combine powdered milk, baking soda and cornstarch.

2. Cover the jar and shake to mix well.

3. Add the essential oils, cover and shake the jar again to combine.

4. Set aside to cure for at least 24 hours

5. Usage: Pour 1 or 2 cups of the milk bath directly under running bath water. Disperse with your hands to mix.

6. Slide into the water and relax for 20 to 30 minutes.

7. Finish up by applying body oil or a hydrating lotion.

Caution: Do not use chamomile if you are allergic to ragweed.

Sunshine Citrus Milk Bath

Ingredients:

2 cups of whole powdered milk

1/4 cup baking soda

1/2 cup cornstarch

10 drops bergamot essential oil

9 drops orange essential oil

1 drop rose geranium or jasmine essential oil

Directions:

1. In a dark glass jar, combine powdered milk, baking soda and cornstarch.

2. Cover the jar and shake to mix well.

3. Add the essential oils, cover and shake the jar again to combine.

4. Set aside to cure for at least 24 hours

5. Usage: Pour 1 or 2 cups of the milk bath directly under running bath water. Disperse with your hands to mix.

6. Slide into the water and relax for 20 to 30 minutes.

7. Finish up by applying body oil or a hydrating lotion.

Caution: Do not use prior to sun exposure because orange and bergamot may cause sunburn.

Spicy And Silky Milk Bath

Ingredients:

2 cups of whole powdered milk

1/4 cup baking soda

1/2 cup cornstarch

10 drops lavender essential oil

9 drops sandalwood essential oil

1 drop clove essential oil

Directions:

1. In a dark glass jar, combine powdered milk, baking soda and cornstarch.

2. Cover the jar and shake to mix well.

3. Add the essential oils, cover and shake the jar again to combine.

4. Set aside to cure for at least 24 hours

5. Usage: Pour 1 or 2 cups of the milk bath directly under running bath water. Disperse with your hands to mix.

6. Slide into the water and relax for 20 to 30 minutes.

7. Finish up by applying body oil or a hydrating lotion.

Caution: Leave out clove if you have sensitive skin.

Sweet Haven Milk Bath

Ingredients:

2 cups of whole powdered milk

1/4 cup baking soda

1/2 cup cornstarch

12 drops of vanilla absolute essential oil

Directions:

1. In a dark glass jar, combine powdered milk, baking soda and cornstarch.

2. Cover the jar and shake to mix well.

3. Add the essential oil, cover and shake the jar again to combine.

4. Set aside to cure for at least 24 hours

5. Usage: Pour 1 or 2 cups of the milk bath directly under running bath water. Disperse with your hands to mix.

6. Slide into the water and relax for 20 to 30 minutes.

7. Finish up by applying body oil or a hydrating lotion.

Rose Absolute Milk Bath

Ingredients:

2 cups of whole powdered milk

1/4 cup baking soda

1/2 cup cornstarch

6 drops rose absolute essential oil

3 drops palmarosa essential oil

1 drop rose geranium essential oil

Directions:

1. In a dark glass jar, combine powdered milk, baking soda and cornstarch.

2. Cover the jar and shake to mix well.

3. Add the essential oil, cover and shake the jar again to combine.

4. Set aside to cure for at least 24 hours

5. Usage: Pour 1 or 2 cups of the milk bath directly under running bath water. Disperse with your hands to mix.

6. Slide into the water and relax for 20 to 30 minutes.

7. Finish up by applying body oil or a hydrating lotion.

SHOWER STEAMER RECIPES

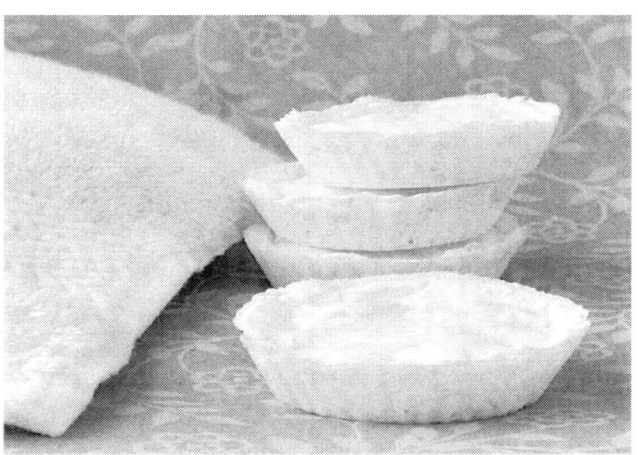

Turn Shower Time To Fun Time

If you like having fun in the bathroom, these are lovely products you should make. They make wonderful gifts too! They are fizzy little gems that everyone will love.

Energizing Shower Steamer

Ingredients:

1 cup citric acid

2 cups baking soda

1 spray bottle of witch hazel

30 drops lemon essential oil

30 drops peppermint essential oil

5 drops basil or geranium essential oil

Directions:

1. Using a fine sieve, sift the citric acid and baking soda pressing to get rid of lumps. Stir together the mixture.

2. Add the essential oils, stirring to combine.

3. Spray some of the witch hazel on the mixture then stir vigorously with your fingers or a fork.

4. Continue spraying and stirring until the mixture binds together when squeezed. However, it should not be wet. It is ready when it holds its shape after being squeezed together with your hands.

5. Press your shower steamer firmly and tightly into molds of your choice (like candy molds or silicone muffin tins). Press it down into the mold so it is tightly packed.

6. Set aside for an hour then flip over each mold and gently tap out the shower steamers onto a flat surface.

7. Now, cover them loosely with a piece of plastic wrap then let them sit for several hours to dry completely.

8. Wrap up the dry shower steamers with parchment paper or plastic wrap and store in an air-tight container.

9. Usage: While taking a shower, place the shower steamer on the floor and let it steam away. It will release a burst of scent each time the spray hits it.

Anti-Stuffiness Shower Steamer

This recipe is good for colds and congestion.

Ingredients:

1 cup citric acid

2 cups baking soda

1 spray bottle of witch hazel

30 drops peppermint essential oil

25 drops eucalyptus essential oil

10 drops tea tree essential oil

Directions:

1. Using a fine sieve, sift the citric acid and baking soda pressing to get rid of lumps. Stir together the mixture.

2. Add the essential oils, stirring to combine.

3. Spray some of the witch hazel on the mixture then stir vigorously with your fingers or a fork.

4. Continue spraying and stirring until the mixture binds together when squeezed. However, it should not be wet. It is ready when it holds its shape after being squeezed together with your hands.

5. Press your shower steamer firmly and tightly into molds of your choice (like candy molds or silicone muffin tins). Press it down into the mold so it is tightly packed.

6. Set aside for an hour then flip over each mold and gently tap out the shower steamers onto a flat surface.

7. Now, cover them loosely with a piece of plastic wrap then let them sit for several hours to dry completely.

8. Wrap up the dry shower steamers with parchment paper or plastic wrap and store in an air-tight container.

9. Usage: While taking a shower, place the shower steamer on the floor and let it steam away. It will release a burst of scent each time the spray hits it.

After Workout Shower Steamer

Ingredients:

1 cup citric acid

2 cups baking soda

1 spray bottle of witch hazel

30 drops grapefruit essential oil

25 drops lavender essential oil

10 drops peppermint essential oil

Directions:

1. Using a fine sieve, sift the citric acid and baking soda pressing to get rid of lumps. Stir together the mixture.

2. Add the essential oils, stirring to combine.

3. Spray some of the witch hazel on the mixture then stir vigorously with your fingers or a fork.

4. Continue spraying and stirring until the mixture binds together when squeezed. However, it should not be wet. It is ready when it holds its shape after being squeezed together with your hands.

5. Press your shower steamer firmly and tightly into molds of your choice (like candy molds or silicone muffin tins). Press it down into the mold so it is tightly packed.

6. Set aside for an hour then flip over each mold and gently tap out the shower steamers onto a flat surface.

7. Now, cover them loosely with a piece of plastic wrap then let them sit for several hours to dry completely.

8. Wrap up the dry shower steamers with parchment paper or plastic wrap and store in an air-tight container.

9. Usage: While taking a shower, place the shower steamer on the floor and let it steam away. It will release a burst of scent each time the spray hits it.

Uplifting Shower Steamer

Use this when you are cranky or depressed.

Ingredients:

1 cup citric acid

2 cups baking soda

1 spray bottle of witch hazel

25 drops lavender essential oil

30 drops bergamot, grapefruit or lemon essential oil

5 drops frankincense essential oil

3 drops rosemary essential oil

2 drops geranium essential oil

Directions:

1. Using a fine sieve, sift the citric acid and baking soda pressing to get rid of lumps. Stir together the mixture.

2. Add the essential oils, stirring to combine.

3. Spray some of the witch hazel on the mixture then stir vigorously with your fingers or a fork.

4. Continue spraying and stirring until the mixture binds together when squeezed. However, it should not be wet. It is ready when it holds its shape after being squeezed together with your hands.

5. Press your shower steamer firmly and tightly into molds of your choice (like candy molds or silicone muffin tins). Press it down into the mold so it is tightly packed.

6. Set aside for an hour then flip over each mold and gently tap out the shower steamers onto a flat surface.

7. Now, cover them loosely with a piece of plastic wrap then let them sit for several hours to dry completely.

8. Wrap up the dry shower steamers with parchment paper or plastic wrap and store in an air-tight container.

9. Usage: While taking a shower, place the shower steamer on the floor and let it steam away. It will release a burst of scent each time the spray hits it.

Relaxing Shower Steamer

Use this to beat insomnia and have a restful night.

Ingredients:

1 cup citric acid

2 cups baking soda

1 spray bottle of witch hazel

30 drops lavender essential oil

15 drops frankincense essential oil

15 drops sandalwood essential oil

3 drops vetiver essential oil

2 drops geranium essential oil

Directions:

1. Using a fine sieve, sift the citric acid and baking soda pressing to get rid of lumps. Stir together the mixture.

2. Add the essential oils, stirring to combine.

3. Spray some of the witch hazel on the mixture then stir vigorously with your fingers or a fork.

4. Continue spraying and stirring until the mixture binds together when squeezed. However, it should not be wet. It is ready when it holds its shape after being squeezed together with your hands.

5. Press your shower steamer firmly and tightly into molds of your choice (like candy molds or silicone muffin tins). Press it down into the mold so it is tightly packed.

6. Set aside for an hour then flip over each mold and gently tap out the shower steamers onto a flat surface.

7. Now, cover them loosely with a piece of plastic wrap then let them sit for several hours to dry completely.

8. Wrap up the dry shower steamers with parchment paper or plastic wrap and store in an air-tight container.

9. Usage: While taking a shower, place the shower steamer on the floor and let it steam away. It will release a burst of scent each time the spray hits it.

Spicy Shower Steamer

Ingredients:

1 cup citric acid

2 cups baking soda

1 spray bottle of witch hazel

35 drops lavender essential oil

25 drops patchouli essential oil

5 drops clove essential oil

Directions:

1. Using a fine sieve, sift the citric acid and baking soda pressing to get rid of lumps. Stir together the mixture.

2. Add the essential oils, stirring to combine.

3. Spray some of the witch hazel on the mixture then stir vigorously with your fingers or a fork.

4. Continue spraying and stirring until the mixture binds together when squeezed. However, it should not be wet. It is ready when it holds its shape after being squeezed together with your hands.

5. Press your shower steamer firmly and tightly into molds of your choice (like candy molds or silicone muffin tins). Press it down into the mold so it is tightly packed.

6. Set aside for an hour then flip over each mold and gently tap out the shower steamers onto a flat surface.

7. Now, cover them loosely with a piece of plastic wrap then let them sit for several hours to dry completely.

8. Wrap up the dry shower steamers with parchment paper or plastic wrap and store in an air-tight container.

9. Usage: While taking a shower, place the shower steamer on the floor and let it steam away. It will release a burst of scent each time the spray hits it.

BODY BUTTER RECIPES

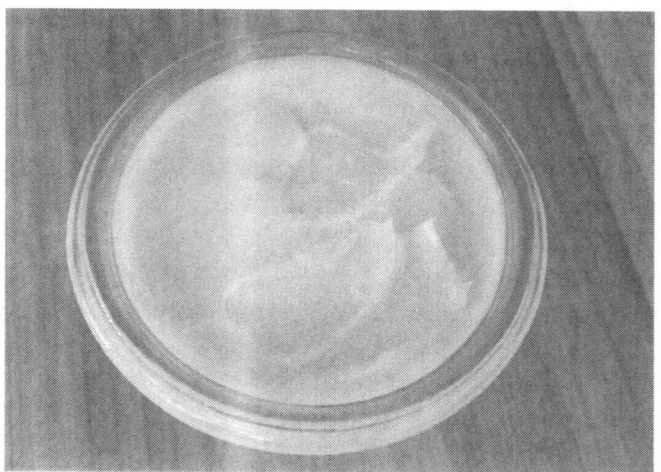

Save Your skin With Wearable Vitamins

These yummy recipes below will help you to make your own lovely aromatherapy body butter. They are creamy, deeply moisturizing and rich in minerals, vitamins and emollients. When you use natural body butters, your skin stays hydrated for a longer period because the cream forms a protective barrier that locks in moisture. They are great for individuals with dry, chapped, wind-burned or cracked skin. You can also use then for sensual massage with your partner.

One of the secrets to natural body butters is to choose the ideal base for your skin type.

Cocoa Butter - This butter is unique because it has the ability to slow down the production of immuno globulin IgE and this helps to reduce the symptoms of asthma and dermatitis. By creating a barrier between your skin and the environment, moisture is retained, you are protected from wind or sun damage and wrinkles and stretch marks are reduced. Recipes that have cocoa butter have also been shown by researchers to boost the immune system, relieve stress and prevent cancer.

Shea Butter - Has a lot of vitamins, antioxidants and essential fatty acids. It improves elasticity, reduces wrinkles and helps to heal sores, burns, scars, dandruff, psoriasis, eczema and stretch marks. Not recommended if you have nut or latex allergies.

Mango Butter - Moisturizing and soothing mango butter protects your skin against UV radiation. It is good for healing psoriasis, eczema, bug bites, rashes, frostbite, sunburn, stretch marks, cracked skin and more. Many dermatologists recommend it for reducing wrinkles.

Home Spa Sensual Body Butter Massage Cream

This rich honey sweetened body butter is excellent for silky-smooth skin and sensual massage.

Makes about 8 ounces

Ingredients:

3/4 cup Shea butter

3/4 cup cocoa butter

2 tablespoons jojoba or apricot kernel oil

1 capsule vitamin E (or 1/4 teaspoon)

8 drops lavender essential oil

8 drops palmarosa essential oil

8 drops rose essential oil

2 drops clary sage essential oil

2 drops rose geranium essential oil

Directions:

1. Melt Shea butter and cocoa butter in a double boiler on low heat, about 20 minutes.

2. Remove from the heat then add the oil and vitamin E, stirring with a metal spoon to combine.

3. Set the bowl of body butter in a larger bowl of ice water so that it can cool faster. Now add the essential oils.

4. Whip the butter with an electric hand mixer continually for several minutes until fluffy. Repeat every 10 minutes until you have the desired consistency.

5. Spoon the body butter into a dark glass jar.

6. Apply a generous amount of the body butter to damp skin immediately after a bath or shower.

Deluxe Lavender Body Butter

Heal dry and cracked skin with this lush aromatherapy body butter recipe that will moisturize deeply and nourish. The added essential oils enhance the growth of healthy skin cells. Good for dry, aging skin, psoriasis and eczema.

Makes about 8 ounces

Ingredients:

1 cup Shea butter

1/4 cup cocoa butter

1 tablespoon rosehip oil

1 tablespoon jojoba oil

2 tablespoons sweet almond oil

1 capsule vitamin E (or 1/4 teaspoon)

1 teaspoon corn starch (for reducing greasiness)

20 drops lavender essential oil

4 drops sandalwood essential oil

4 drops patchouli essential oil

2 drops cedarwood essential oil

Directions:

1. Melt Shea butter and cocoa butter in a double boiler on low heat, about 20 minutes.

2. Remove from the heat then add the oils, vitamin E and corn starch, stirring with a metal spoon to combine.

3. Set the bowl of body butter in a larger bowl of ice water so that it can cool faster. Now add the essential oils.

4. Whip the butter with an electric hand mixer continually for several minutes until fluffy. Repeat every 10 minutes until you have the desired consistency.

5. Spoon the body butter into a dark glass jar.

6. Apply a generous amount of the body butter to damp skin immediately after a bath or shower.

Sunshine Mango Cirtrus Body Butter

Cheer yourself up with this sparkling body butter with a divine scent. It is suitable for all types of skin. Good for stretch marks, cracked skin, wrinkles, psoriasis and eczema. It will also nourish your skin deeply and sooth your nerves.

Makes about 8 ounces

Ingredients:

1/3 cup mango butter

2/3 cup Shea butter

3 teaspoons grapeseed oil

1 teaspoon jojoba oil

1 capsule vitamin E (or 1/4 teaspoon)

10 drops bergamot essential oil

8 drops palmarosa essential oil

8 drops lemongrass essential oil

1 drop ylang ylang essential oil

2 drops cypress essential oil

1 teaspoon corn starch (for reducing greasiness)

Cosmetic mica (optional – for glitter)

Directions:

1. Melt mango butter and Shea butter in a double boiler on low heat, about 20 minutes.

2. Remove from the heat then add the oils, vitamin E, cosmetic mica and corn starch, stirring with a metal spoon to combine.

3. Set the bowl of body butter in a larger bowl of ice water so that it can cool faster. Now add the essential oils.

4. Whip the butter with an electric hand mixer continually for several minutes until fluffy. Repeat every 10 minutes until you have the desired consistency.

5. Spoon the body butter into a dark glass jar.

6. Apply a generous amount of the body butter to damp skin immediately after a bath or shower.

Organic Vanilla Body Cream

Makes about 4 ounces of cream

Ingredients:

2 tablespoons Shea butter

4 tablespoons sweet almond oil

2 tablespoons virgin coconut oil

1/2 teaspoon pure vanilla absolute essential oil

Directions:

1. Melt the Shea butter in a double boiler on low heat.

2. Combine the melted Shea with the other ingredients in a food processor and blend together.

3. Scoop into a dark colored glass jar. Can be kept in the refrigerator for up to 4 months.

BODY SCRUB RECIPES

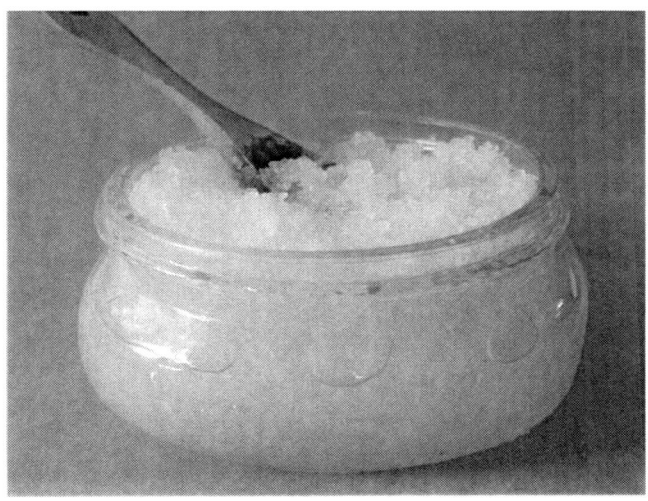

Exfoliating Body Treatments

It is easy to make your own body scrubs that will make your skin smooth and silky. These exfoliating treatments are designed to remove the roughness, dead skin, unclog pores and leave you with soft and smooth skin. Additionally, they detoxify the body, stimulate the circulation of blood and lymph, and help to fight cellulite. Exfoliating is vital if you are battling acne. Endeavor to exfoliate at least once a week with a homemade body scrub. Using a body scrub prior to other skin treatments opens up the pores and enables other products to work more effectively. You can use a Salt Scrub, Sugar Scrub, Loofa Scrub or Fruit Scrub. Do not use body scrubs if your sin is fragile, sunburned, broken, or if you have certain allergies.

Peppermint-Citrus Salt Scrub

This is a refreshing body scrub that smoothens, cleanses and stimulates your skin. It is useful for balancing oil production in normal, combination or oily and acne-prone skin.

Ingredients:

1/2 cup sea salt

2 tablespoons grapeseed or any other carrier oil

1 1/2 teaspoons Aloe Vera gel

2 drops rosemary essential oil

5 drops peppermint essential oil

8 drops orange essential oil

Directions:

1. Combine salt, oil and Aloe Vera gel in a ceramic or glass bowl. Stir together with a metal spoon.

2. Add the essential oils and stir until well combined.

3. Usage: Take a warm shower but do not dry your body. Stand in the bathtub and rub the body scrub with gentle circular motions all over your skin.

4. Rinse off with water, dry your body with a towel and moisturize.

Caution: Do not use salt based body scrubs if your skin is irritated or broken. Avoid face and genitals. Do not use prior to sun exposure because the sweet orange essential oil may cause sunburn.

Chamomile And Oatmeal Body Scrub

Recommended for dry, mature, sensitive or damaged skin. It removes flaky skin, nourishes, calms irritation and restores moisture.

Ingredients:

1/4 cup of rolled oats, ground fine

1/4 cup of almonds, ground fine

1 tablespoon sweet almond oil

2 drops chamomile essential oil

4 drops rosewood essential oil

9 drops palmarosa essential oil

Directions:

1. Using a clean coffee grinder and working in separate batches, grind the oats and almonds until you get a fine texture.

2. Combine ground oats, ground almond and sweet almond oil in a ceramic or glass bowl and stir together with a metal spoon.

3. Add the essential oils and stir until well combined.

4. Usage: Take a warm shower but do not dry your body. Stand in the bathtub and rub the body scrub with gentle circular motions all over your skin.

5. Rinse off with water, dry your body with a towel and moisturize.

Brown Sugar Vanilla Body Scrub

Good for all types of skin. This soothing body scrub can be used on fragile skin and also for conditions like eczema and psoriasis. Regular use can also lead to the reduction of fine lines and wrinkles.

Ingredients:

1/2 cup brown sugar

2 tablespoons of sweet almond oil or any other carrier oil

1 drop ylang ylang essential oil

4 drops sandalwood essential oil

10 drops vanilla absolute essential oil

Directions:

1. Combine brown sugar and sweet almond oil in a ceramic or glass bowl. Stir together with a metal spoon.

2. Add the essential oils and stir until well combined.

3. Usage: Take a warm shower but do not dry your body. Stand in the bathtub and rub the body scrub with gentle circular motions all over your skin.

4. If your bathroom is warm, leave it on your skin to dry and tighten for a few minutes.

5. Rinse off with water, dry your body with a towel and moisturize.

Caution: Do not use salt based body scrubs if your skin is irritated or broken. Avoid face and genitals.

Yogurt And Honey Body Scrub

Good for irritated, sensitive or problematic skin.

Ingredients:

1/4 cup of rolled oats, ground fine

1/4 cup of wheat bran

1/2 cup full fat yogurt

1 tablespoon honey

1 tablespoon of sweet almond oil

2 drops chamomile essential oil

2 drops rose essential oil

3 drops palmarosa essential oil

8 drops lavender essential oil

Directions:

1. Using a clean coffee grinder, grind the oats until you get a fine texture.

2. Combine ground oats and wheat bran in a ceramic or glass bowl and stir together with a metal spoon.

3. In a medium-sized bowl, stir together the honey, yogurt and sweet almond oil. Add the oats mixture as well as the essential oils. Stir the mixture properly to combine.

4. Usage: Take a warm shower but do not dry your body. Stand in the bathtub and rub the body scrub with gentle circular motions all over your skin.

5. Rinse off with water, dry your body with a towel and moisturize.

Caution: Do not use salt based body scrubs if your skin is irritated or broken. Avoid face and genitals. For individuals with ragweed allergies, use 3 drops of lavender essential oil in place of chamomile.

Coffee Body Scrub

An inexpensive cellulite treatment to deep-cleanse pores, removing excess water from the skin and promote circulation.

Ingredients:

1 cup of fresh-ground coffee

1/2 cup coconut oil

1/2 cup salt

1/2 cup brown sugar

Directions:

1. Mix together all the ingredients.

2. Using a circular motion, massage into cellulite-prone areas like the butt, thighs, hips and stomach.

3. Keep massaging for about 5 minutes then rinse.

Repeat 3-5 times every week.

DIY LOTION RECIPES

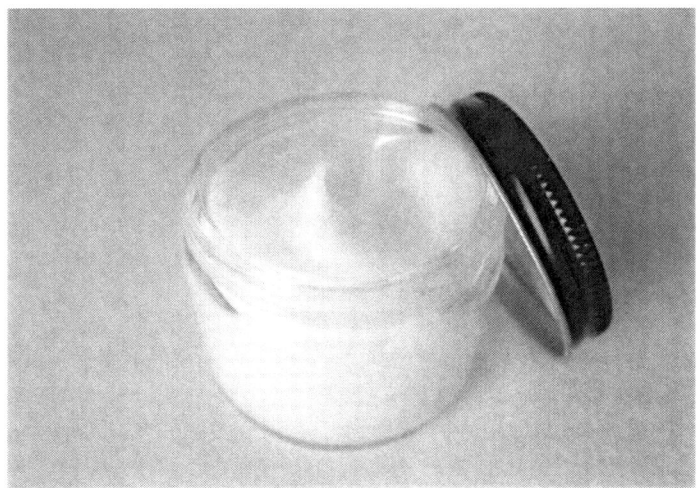

Pamper Your Skin with Homemade Natural Lotions

Using natural moisturizers is vital to having healthy skin. They make it easy to provide your skin with the needed nourishment, healing and strength. The recipes in this section are not only effective, they are also inexpensive and you will have fun making them.

Lush Lavender DIY Body Lotion

Lavender has a lot of valuable properties that will help you to have great skin.

Makes about 8 ounces

Ingredients:

2 tablespoons emulsifying wax

2 tablespoons vegetable glycerin

1/2 teaspoon stearic acid

1/3 cup grapeseed or jojoba oil

1/2 cup of distilled water

1 teaspoon vitamin E

10 drops grapefruit seed extract

2 drops cedarwood essential oil

8 drops sandalwood essential oil

20 drops lavender essential oil

Directions:

1. Stir together emulsifying wax, glycerin, stearic acid and oil. Melt the mixture in a double boiler over low heat.

2. Remove from heat and add Vitamin E.

3. In the microwave or in another pot on your stove, warm water until just lukewarm.

4. Pour the water slowly into the oil, constantly stirring with a wire whisk until you have a thick and smooth mixture.

5. Stir in the grapefruit seed extract and the essential oils.

6. Transfer the lotion into an 8oz dark glass bottle and let it cool before covering with the lid. Occasionally shake the bottle as the mixture cools so the ingredients will not separate.

7. Store in a cool and dark place.

Spicy Peppermint DIY Body Lotion

This cool, minty moisturizer is good for oily skin, itchy skin and sunburned skin. Besides nourishing and replenishing moisture, it also heals bites and burns.

Makes about 8 ounces

Ingredients:

2 tablespoons emulsifying wax

1 tablespoon vegetable glycerin

1/3 cup grapeseed oil

1/2 cup peppermint floral water or distilled water

1 teaspoon vitamin E

2 drops palmarosa essential oil

10 drops grapefruit seed extract

10 drops lavender essential oil

18 drops peppermint essential oil

Directions:

1. Stir together emulsifying wax, glycerin and oil. Melt the mixture in a double boiler over low heat.

2. Remove from heat and add Vitamin E.

3. In the microwave or in another pot on your stove, warm water or floral water until just lukewarm.

4. Pour the water slowly into the oil, constantly stirring with a wire whisk until you have a thick and smooth mixture.

5. Stir in the grapefruit seed extract and the essential oils.

6. Transfer the lotion into an 8oz dark glass bottle and let it cool before covering with the lid. Occasionally shake the bottle as the mixture cools so the ingredients will not separate.

7. Store in a cool and dark place.

Exotic DIY Body Lotion

This rich and creamy lotion, hydrates, soothes and heals damaged and dry skin. It is great when your hands and feet are chapped by harsh weather. It also has a scent that men will love.

Makes about 8 ounces

Ingredients:

2 tablespoons emulsifying wax

2 tablespoons vegetable glycerin

1/3 cup apricot kernel or jojoba oil

1/2 cup of distilled water

1 teaspoon vitamin E

20 drops sandalwood essential oil

10 drops grapefruit seed extract

5 drops frankincense essential oil

5 drops patchouli essential oil

Directions:

1. Stir together emulsifying wax, glycerin and oil. Melt the mixture in a double boiler over low heat.

2. Remove from heat and add Vitamin E.

3. In the microwave or in another pot on your stove, warm water until just lukewarm.

4. Pour the water slowly into the oil, constantly stirring with a wire whisk until you have a thick and smooth mixture.

5. Stir in the grapefruit seed extract and the essential oils.

6. Transfer the lotion into an 8oz dark glass bottle and let it cool before covering with the lid. Occasionally shake the bottle as the mixture cools so the ingredients will not separate.

7. Store in a cool and dark place.

Minty Aloe DIY Sunscreen

Making your own sunscreen enables you to know exactly what goes into it. Now you can avoid buying store brand sunscreens that contain many ingredients that are not good for your skin.

Makes about 8 ounces

Ingredients:

1 tablespoon of emulsifying wax

2 tablespoons zinc oxide

1/3 cup grapeseed or jojoba oil

1 teaspoon vitamin E

1/2 cup distilled water

2 tablespoons Aloe Vera gel

10 drops peppermint essential oil

10 drops spearmint essential oil

10 drops grapefruit seed extract

1 drop ylang ylang essential oil

5 drops lemongrass essential oil

Directions:

1. Stir together emulsifying wax, oil and zinc oxide. Melt the mixture in a double boiler over low heat.

2. Remove from heat and add Vitamin E.

3. In the microwave or in another pot on your stove, warm water and Aloe vera gel until just lukewarm.

4. Pour the water slowly into the oil, constantly stirring with a wire whisk until you have a thick and smooth mixture.

5. Stir in the grapefruit seed extract and the essential oils.

6. Transfer the lotion into an 8oz dark glass bottle and let it cool before covering with the lid. Occasionally shake the bottle as the mixture cools so the ingredients will not separate.

7. Store in a cool and dark place.

Caution: Wear gloves and use a mask when making this recipe to protect you from inhaling zinc oxide.

DIY Bug Repellent Lotion

The essential oils in this recipe provide effective and natural protection from insects.

Makes about 8 ounces

Ingredients:

2 tablespoons emulsifying wax

1/3 cup grapeseed oil

1/2 teaspoon stearic acid

1 teaspoon vitamin E

1/2 cup lavender floral water or distilled water

10 drops grapefruit seed extract

10 drops lemongrass essential oil

10 drops lemon eucalyptus essential oil

10 drops citronella essential oil

Directions:

1. Stir together emulsifying wax, oil and stearic acid. Melt the mixture in a double boiler over low heat.

2. Remove from heat and add Vitamin E.

3. In the microwave or in another pot on your stove, warm water or lavender floral water until just lukewarm.

4. Pour the water slowly into the oil, constantly stirring with a wire whisk until you have a thick and smooth mixture.

5. Stir in the grapefruit seed extract and the essential oils.

6. Transfer the lotion into an 8oz dark glass bottle and let it cool before covering with the lid. Occasionally shake the bottle as the mixture cools so the ingredients will not separate.

7. Store in a cool and dark place.

8. This natural bug repellent lotion lasts up to 6 hours on your skin.

Vanilla Massage Oil Lotion Bar

Make your skin silky-sweet with this rich and sensual lotion bar. It is also an edible body butter.

Makes about 4 ounces

Ingredients:

1 tablespoon grated cocoa butter

3 tablespoons shea butter

2 tablespoons of virgin coconut oil

2 tablespoons of sweet almond oil

1 capsule vitamin E (or 1/4 teaspoon)

1 teaspoon of honey powder

6 drops of vanilla absolute essential oil

Directions:

1. Melt Shea butter, cocoa butter and coconut oil in a double boiler on low heat, about 20 minutes.

2. Stir in the almond oil then remove from heat.

3. Now add the vitamin E, vanilla essential oil and honey powder, whisking to combine.

4. Pour the mixture into a silicone muffin tin or small-size silicone soap molds.

5. Let cool for about 2 hours then pop out (you may place in the fridge for a few minutes before popping it out of the mold).

6. Wrap in plastic wrap or parchment paper until you want to use

Exotic Shea Butter Lotion Bar

This lotion nourishes deeply and its soothing and healing properties are good for hydrating, dry and cracked skin.

Ingredients:

3/4 cup shea butter

3/4 cup cocoa butter

3/4 cup of beeswax

3/4 cup of unrefined coconut oil

5 drops grapefruit seed extract

1 capsule vitamin E (or 1/4 teaspoon)

10 drops sandalwood essential oil

8 drops patchouli essential oil

8 drops orange essential oil

1 drop cinnamon essential oil

1 drop ginger essential oil

1 drop vetiver essential oil

Directions:

1. Melt Shea butter, cocoa butter, beeswax and coconut oil in a double boiler on low heat, about 10 minutes.

2. Remove from heat and add grapefruit seed extract, Vitamin E and essential oils then use a metal spoon to stir together thoroughly.

3. Pour the mixture into a silicone muffin tin or small-size silicone soap molds.

4. Let cool for about 2 hours then pop out (you may place in the fridge for a few minutes before popping it out of the mold).

5. Wrap in plastic wrap or parchment paper until you want to use.

Chocolate Peppermint Lotion Bars

These not only smell delicious, they also moisturize the skin very well.

Ingredients:

1/2 cup cocoa butter

1/2 cup beeswax

1/2 cup of coconut oil

2 teaspoons of peppermint essential oil

Directions:

1. Melt cocoa butter, beeswax and coconut oil in a double boiler on low heat.

2. Remove from heat and let cool for some minutes.

3. Add the peppermint essential oil, stirring it in with a wooden skewer.

4. Pour into molds and let cool completely on the counter. For faster cooling, you may place in the freezer for 30 minutes.

Homemade Solid Lotion Bar

This lotion bar is recommended for dry skin.

Ingredients:

1/2 cup Shea butter

1 tablespoon jojoba wax spheres

1/2 cup beeswax (refined beads)

1/2 cup jojoba oil

2 to 4 teaspoons essential oil

Directions:

1. Melt the Shea butter then pour it into a 16-ounce Pyrex measuring cup.

2. Add the jojoba wax spheres and beeswax then melt in the microwave.

3. Add the jojoba oil, mix well. Let cool slightly then add the essential oil.

4. Pour the mixture into small-size soap molds. Let cool for about 2 hours then pop out (you may place in the fridge for a few minutes before popping it out of the mold).

AROMATHERAPY MASSAGE OIL RECIPES

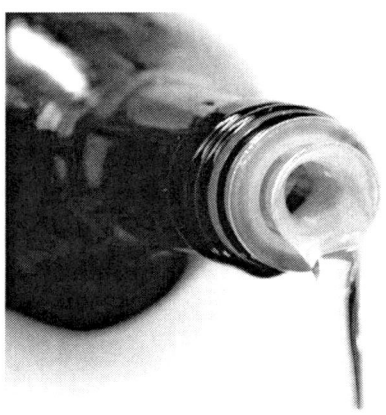

Pamper Your Body With Aromatherapy Massage

These massage oils are relaxing and you can make them any time you like. They provide lubrication and help your skin to retain moisture. When used for massage, the oils are absorbed easily by skin tissues to supply therapeutic skin conditioning.

Blissful Citrus Homemade Massage Oil

This uplifting massage oil provides the perfect remedy for depression.

Ingredients:

15 drops of bergamot essential oil

15 drops of palmarosa essential oil

2 drops of ylang ylang essential oil

1/4 cup of jojoba oil apricot kernel oil

Directions:

1. Mix together all the ingredients in a dark glass bottle.

2. Set aside to cure for at least 24 hours in a cool dark place.

3. Use it for a full body massage.

4. Last up to 3 months.

Caution: Do not use prior to sun exposure because the bergamot essential oil may cause sunburn.

Lavender Aromatherapy Massage Oil

Pretty and beautifully scented lavender provides healing for the body in a variety of ways.

Ingredients:

12 drops of lavender essential oil

12 drops of orange essential oil

2 drops clary sage essential oil

3 drops marjoram essential oil

1 drop of vetiver essential oil

1/4 cup jojoba oil or sweet almond oil

Directions:

1. Mix together all the ingredients in a dark glass bottle.

2. Set aside to cure for at least 24 hours in a cool dark place.

3. Use it for a full body massage or rub it on your chest, stomach and feet just before bed for a restful night.

4. Last up to 3 months.

Caution: Do not use prior to sun exposure because the orange essential oil may cause sunburn.

Lavender Therapeutic Massage Oil

Use this when you have a throbbing headache, sore muscles, sore joints or an aching back. It will reduce inflammation, soothe your nerves and relax tight muscles

Ingredients:

8 drops of lavender essential oil

4 drops of marjoram essential oil

1 drop ginger essential oil

1 drop chamomile essential oil

1 drop cedarwood essential oil

1/4 cup jojoba oil or apricot kernel oil

Directions:

1. Mix together all the ingredients in a dark glass bottle.

2. Set aside to cure for at least 24 hours in a cool dark place.

3. Use it for a full body massage.

4. Last up to 3 months.

Caution: Do not use ginger if your skin is exceptionally sensitive. Also leave out the chamomile if you are allergic to ragweed.

Marjoram Anti-Snoring Massage Oil

This recipe has ingredients with sedative properties that support breathing and helps the respiratory system to relax. Even if you do not snore, you can use it for a more relaxed sleep.

Ingredients:

4 drops marjoram essential oil

8 drops lavender essential oil

3 drops lemon essential oil

1/4 cup of apricot kernel oil or sunflower oil

Directions:

1. Mix together all the ingredients in a dark glass bottle.

2. Set aside to cure for at least 24 hours in a cool dark place.

3. Usage: Rub the massage oil gently on the neck, upper chest and behind the ears.

4. Last up to 3 months.

Caution: Do not use prior to sun exposure because the lemon essential oil may cause sunburn.

Stress Relief Aromatherapy Massage Oil

This is a great remedy to bring relief to your body after a hectic day. It is good for days when you feel overwhelmed by the tasks you have to do.

Ingredients:

5 drops frankincense essential oil

5 drops petitgrain essential oil

3 drops marjoram essential oil

1 drop vetiver essential oil

1 drop jasmine essential oil

1/4 cup jojoba oil or apricot kernel oil

Directions:

1. Mix together all the ingredients in a dark glass bottle.

2. Set aside to cure for at least 24 hours in a cool dark place.

3. Use it for a full body massage or rub it on your chest, stomach and feet just before bed for a restful night. You may also rub it on your temple during break time at work.

4. Last up to 3 months.

Sweet And Spicy Aphrodisiac Massage Oil

Use this sensual massage oil when you want to have a nice night in with your partner.

Ingredients:

8 drops of sandalwood essential oil

2 drops patchouli essential oil

3 drops orange essential oil

1 drop ginger essential oil

1 drop ylang ylang essential oil

1/4 cup jojoba oil or apricot kernel oil

Directions:

1. Mix together all the ingredients in a dark glass bottle.

2. Set aside to cure for at least 24 hours in a cool dark place.

3. Usage: Use it for a full body massage or heat the bottle in a bowl of hot water and then have a hot oil massage.

4. Last up to 3 months.

Caution: Do not use ginger if your skin is exceptionally sensitive. Do not use prior to sun exposure because the lemon essential oil may cause sunburn.

ESSENTIAL OILS PERFUME RECIPES

Make Your Own Signature Scent

Aromatherapy perfume recipes come in various beautiful fragrances and you can find one for every mood. They smell fabulous, uplift your mood, boost the immune system, calm your nerves and more!

Mystifying Aromatherapy Perfume

Ingredients:

8 drops sandalwood essential oil

3 drops lavender essential oil

1 drop cedarwood essential oil

1 tablespoon vodka

1 tablespoon grapeseed or jojoba oil

Directions:

1. Using a funnel, pour the alcohol and carrier oil into a 2oz dark glass bottle.

2. Drop in all the essential oils.

3. Cover the bottle then shake it to mix well.

4. Keep the bottle in a cool and dark place for 7-10 days to cure. Shake it several times daily.

5. Apply to pulse points on the sternum, wrist, base of the neck and behind the knees.

Romantic Floral Aromatherapy Perfume

Ingredients:

6 drops palmarosa essential oil

3 drop rose geranium essential oil

1 drop ylang ylang essential oil

1 tablespoon vodka

1 tablespoon grapeseed or jojoba oil

Directions:

1. Using a funnel, pour the alcohol and carrier oil into a 2oz dark glass bottle.

2. Drop in all the essential oils.

3. Cover the bottle then shake it to mix well.

4. Keep the bottle in a cool and dark place for 7-10 days to cure. Shake it several times daily.

5. Apply to pulse points on the sternum, wrist, base of the neck and behind the knees.

Energetic Aromatherapy Perfume

Use this when you want to feel and look younger.

Ingredients:

9 drops grapefruit essential oil

1 drop rose geranium essential oil

1 drop ylang ylang essential oil

1 tablespoon vodka

1 tablespoon grapeseed or jojoba oil

Directions:

1. Using a funnel, pour the alcohol and carrier oil into a 2oz dark glass bottle.

2. Drop in all the essential oils.

3. Cover the bottle then shake it to mix well.

4. Keep the bottle in a cool and dark place for 7-10 days to cure. Shake it several times daily.

5. Apply to pulse points on the sternum, wrist, base of the neck and behind the knees.

Luxurious Lavender Aromatherapy Perfume

Ingredients:

6 drops lavender essential oil

4 drops frankincense essential oil

1 drop rose geranium essential oil

1 tablespoon vodka

1 tablespoon grapeseed or jojoba oil

Directions:

1. Using a funnel, pour the alcohol and carrier oil into a 2oz dark glass bottle.

2. Drop in all the essential oils.

3. Cover the bottle then shake it to mix well.

4. Keep the bottle in a cool and dark place for 7-10 days to cure. Shake it several times daily.

5. Apply to pulse points on the sternum, wrist, base of the neck and behind the knees.

Spicy And Sensual Aromatherapy Perfume

Ingredients:

8 drops sandalwood essential oil

2 drops orange essential oil

1 drop patchouli essential oil

1 drop ylang ylang essential oil

1 tablespoon vodka

1 tablespoon grapeseed or jojoba oil

Directions:

1. Using a funnel, pour the alcohol and carrier oil into a 2oz dark glass bottle.

2. Drop in all the essential oils.

3. Cover the bottle then shake it to mix well.

4. Keep the bottle in a cool and dark place for 7-10 days to cure. Shake it several times daily.

5. Apply to pulse points on the sternum, wrist, base of the neck and behind the knees.

Sweet And Yummy Aromatherapy Perfume

Ingredients:

5 drops vanilla essential oil

4 drops cocoa absolute essential oil

1 drop ylang ylang essential oil

1 tablespoon vodka

1 tablespoon grapeseed or jojoba oil

Directions:

1. Using a funnel, pour the alcohol and carrier oil into a 2oz dark glass bottle.

2. Drop in all the essential oils.

3. Cover the bottle then shake it to mix well.

4. Keep the bottle in a cool and dark place for 7-10 days to cure. Shake it several times daily.

5. Apply to pulse points on the sternum, wrist, base of the neck and behind the knees.

Uplifting Aromatherapy Perfume

Ingredients:

5 drops bergamot essential oil

5 drops grapefruit essential oil

1 drop rose geranium essential oil

1 tablespoon vodka

1 tablespoon grapeseed or jojoba oil

Directions:

1. Using a funnel, pour the alcohol and carrier oil into a 2oz dark glass bottle.

2. Drop in all the essential oils.

3. Cover the bottle then shake it to mix well.

4. Keep the bottle in a cool and dark place for 7-10 days to cure. Shake it several times daily.

5. Apply to pulse points on the sternum, wrist, base of the neck and behind the knees.

AROMATHERAPY DEODORIZING BODY POWDER RECIPES

Body powders are very useful for reducing body odor and controlling sweat throughout the day. These powders absorb excess sweat and the essential oils combat the effect of bacteria that cause odor. You can use them on your feet too. Try the recipes in this section to find out the ones that work best for you.

Simple Deodorant Powder Recipe

Remove body odor and naturally with this recipe.

Ingredients:

1/2 cup of arrowroot powder

2 tablespoons of white cosmetic clay

10 drops petitgrain essential oil

10 drops cypress essential oil

10 drops lavender essential oil

Directions:

1. Mix together the cosmetic clay and arrowroot.

2. Drop in the essential oils gradually and use your fingers to mix well as you go.

3. Store in a container and cover the lid tightly. Let it sit for 2 days before use.

4. Apply with your fingers or a powder puff.

Aromatic Lavender Dusting Powder

Ingredients:

1 cup of arrowroot powder

1/2 cup of cornstarch

1/4 cup of baking soda

3 tablespoons lavender buds, very finely ground

70 drops lavender essential oil

Directions:

1. Whisk the dry ingredients together in a large bowl.

2. Drop in the essential oils gradually and whisk well as you go. Use your fingers to break any clumps.

3. Transfer to a container and cover tightly.

4. Use the powder after bathing.

Spicy Cinnamon Dusting Powder

Ingredients:

1 1/2 cups arrowroot powder

1/4 cup cosmetic clay

1/8 cup baking soda

2 teaspoon ground cinnamon

2 teaspoon ground nutmeg

30 drops vanilla essential oil

10 drops clove essential oil

20 drops cinnamon essential oil

Directions:

1. Whisk the dry ingredients together in a large bowl.

2. Drop in the essential oils gradually and whisk well as you go. Use your fingers to break any clumps.

3. Transfer to a container and cover tightly.

4. Use the powder after bathing.

Peppermint Refreshing Dusting Powder

Ingredients:

1 1/2 cups cornstarch or arrowroot powder

1/2 cup baking soda

3 tablespoons dried peppermint leaves, very finely ground

20 drops peppermint essential oil

Directions:

1. Whisk the dry ingredients together in a large bowl.

2. Drop in the essential oils gradually and whisk well as you go. Use your fingers to break any clumps.

3. Transfer to a container and cover tightly.

4. Use the powder after bathing.

Aromatic Baby Powder

Ingredients:

1 1/2 cups of arrowroot powder

1/2 cup of baking soda

1/2 cup chamomile, elder flowers or calendula, finely powdered

1/2 cup cornstarch

20 drops lavender or Roman chamomile essential oil

Directions:

1. Whisk the dry ingredients together in a large bowl.

2. Drop in the essential oils gradually and whisk well as you go. Use your fingers to break any clumps.

3. Transfer to a container and cover tightly.

4. Use the powder after bathing.

NATURAL HAND AND NAIL CARE

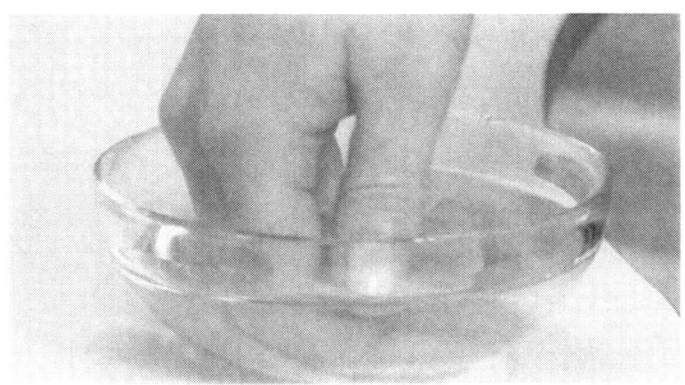

Anti-Aging Hand Oil

Ingredients:

6 tablespoons jojoba oil

2 tablespoons flax seed oil

3 drops carrot seed essential oil

3 drops pomegranate extract

Directions:

1. Mix the ingredients together in a bowl.

2. Apply to your hands then cover with zip lock bags.

3. Leave it on for about 20 minutes then remove and wash hands.

4. Use several times weekly.

Aromatherapy Hand And Foot Soak For Fungus

Ingredients:

1/2 cup warm cider vinegar

6 drops tea tree oil

1/2 cup warm water for hands

** Double the quantities for a foot soak

Directions:

1. In a bowl, combine the ingredients (use a bigger bowl for your feet).

2. Soak for about 10-20 minutes, 4-5 times per week to clear fungus.

Nail Whitener Soak Recipe

Ingredients:

4 tablespoons lemon juice

3 tablespoons warm water

Directions:

1. Mix the water and juice in a ceramic or glass bowl.

2. Soak your nails for about 10 minutes to remove stains.

3. Rinse with water then apply cuticle oil

Nail Growth Soak

Ingredients:

1/4 cup organic coconut oil

1/4 cup organic honey

4 drops rosemary essential oil

Directions:

1. Mix the ingredients together in a bowl.

2. Microwave for 20 seconds to warm.

3. Soak your hands for about 15 minutes.

4. Repeat twice weekly.

Nail Moisturizing Soak

Ingredients:

1 tablespoon of hemp seed Oil

4 drops of lavender essential oil

Directions:

1. Mix the ingredients together in a bowl.

2. Soak your nails for about 15 minutes. Rinse well

NATURAL FOOT CARE

Give Yourself A Foot Lift!

Your feet carry your weight all day and they deserve some pampering now and then. A great way to do this is to make homemade aromatherapy foot scrubs and other recipes that will leave your feet refreshed, soft and smooth.

Spicy Salt Foot Scrub

This foot scrub deodorizes your feet, improves circulation, relieves pain, relaxes your feet and boosts energy.

Ingredients:

1 cup sea salt

4 drops of lavender essential oil

4 drops peppermint essential oil

2 drops black pepper essential oil

1/4 cup olive oil (when you want to use)

2 tablespoons cider vinegar (when you want to use)

Directions:

1. Place the salt in a dark glass jar then add the essential oils.

2. Cap the jar then shake it properly to mix the ingredients.

3. Set aside to cure for at least 24 hours in a cool dark place.

4. Usage: Make a paste by combining 2 tablespoons of the salt/essential oil mixture with water OR 2 tablespoons of cider vinegar.

5. Massage into your feet, giving attention to rough areas.

6. Rinse and dry your feet then apply olive oil.

Sweet And Minty Foot Scrub

This recipe revives and cools aching, tired feet. It also kills odor-producing bacteria and energizes the body.

Ingredients:

1/4 cup Epsom salt or sea salt

1 cup cornmeal

1 drop ylang ylang essential oil

4 drops tea tree essential oil

5 drops peppermint essential oil

2 to 3 tablespoons sweet almond oil (when you want to use)

Directions:

1. Combine salt and cornmeal in a dark glass jar, cover and shake properly.

2. Add the essential oils and shake again.

3. Set aside to cure for at least 24 hours in a cool dark place.

4. Usage: Make a paste by combining 1/4 cup of the foot scrub with water OR 2-3 tablespoons of sweet almond oil.

5. Massage into your feet, giving attention to rough areas.

6. Rinse and dry your feet then apply olive oil.

Avocado Foot Scrub

The abrasiveness of ground avocado pit breaks down calluses, while the oils in the flesh provides nourishment for the skin.

Ingredients:

2 avocados (one ripe one for fruit and the other one for pit)

1/4 cup cornmeal

1 teaspoon sea salt

Directions:

1. Place the avocado in a sunny place to dry for a few days.

2. Use a cooking mallet or hammer to break the dry pit into several pieces.

3. Transfer to a food processor or coffee grinder and grind to form a gritty meal.

4. Scoop out the other avocado and reserve the skin.

5. Mash the avocado fruit together with 1/4 cup of the ground avocado pit, the cornmeal and sea salt.

6. Massage the mixture gently into your feet with a circular motion. Pay attention to the toes and ankle area. Rinse with lukewarm water.

7. Next, take the avocado skin and rub the inside on the heel and other callused areas. Massage for about 5-10 minutes until the abrasiveness wears off. Leave it on for several hours.

Refreshing Foot Soak

This foot soak has a refreshing and pain-relieving effect on aching and tired feet.

Ingredients:

1 cup of baking soda

1/4 cup of borax

1 drop rose geranium essential oil

4 drops eucalyptus essential oil

5 drops peppermint essential oil

1 teaspoon of your preferred carrier oil

Directions:

1. Pour hot water into a large plastic tub (enough for both feet).

2. Add the baking soda and borax then stir to dissolve.

3. If necessary, add some cold water to adjust to a comfortable temperature.

4. In a small bowl, combine the carrier oil and essential oils then add the mixture to the water.

5. Soak your feet in the footbath for 10 to 20 minutes.

6. Rinse, pat dry and moisturize.

Milky Foot Soak

Ingredients:

7 cups water

2 cups milk

2 tablespoon moisturizing lotion

1/2 cup sugar

Directions:

1. Heat the water and milk in a large saucepan.

2. Stir in the lotion and sugar then remove from heat.

3. Pour into a large bowl then allow the mixture to become cool enough for your feet.

4. Soak your feet for 10 minutes.

5. Rinse and apply moisturizer.

NATURAL HAIR CARE

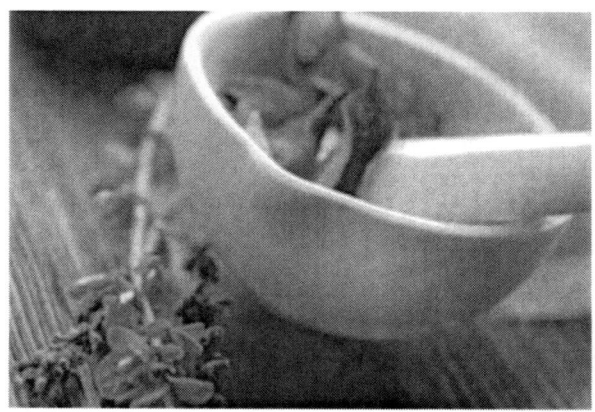

HOMEMADE SHAMPOO RECIPES

Shiny, Soft Hair Naturally

Homemade shampoos are pocket-friendly, healthier and also environmentally friendly. A number of DIY shampoo recipes are provided below. Choose the one that is most suitable for your hair. However, even though you are using natural shampoos, it is not good to wash your hair too frequently so that it will not be stripped of its natural defenses. Washing your hair once every few days is enough and it is advisable to follow each wash with a vinegar hair rinse so as to reduce the buildup of product and to balance the PH.

Dry Hair Homemade Shampoo

Ingredients:

1/2 cup of liquid castile soap

1/2 teaspoon vegetable glycerin

5 drops lavender essential oil

1 drop chamomile essential oil

1 drop clary sage essential oil

1 drop geranium essential oil

1 drop ylang ylang essential oil

Directions:

1. Combine the ingredients in a dark glass bottle.

2. Shake when you want to use. Rinse with cool water.

3. After using the shampoo, use a natural conditioner followed by a vinegar hair rinse.

Oily Hair Homemade Shampoo

Ingredients:

1/2 cup of liquid castile soap

1/2 teaspoon vegetable glycerin

5 drops rosemary essential oil

4 drops juniper essential oil

1 drop cedarwood essential oil

Directions:

1. Combine the ingredients in a dark glass bottle.

2. Shake when you want to use. Rinse with cool water.

3. After using the shampoo, use a natural conditioner followed by a vinegar hair rinse.

Caution: Do not use rosemary essential oil if you have epilepsy or high blood pressure.

Thinning Hair Homemade Shampoo

Ingredients:

1/2 cup of liquid castile soap

1/2 teaspoon vegetable glycerin

5 drops rosemary essential oil

3 drops peppermint essential oil

2 drops bay essential oil

Directions:

1. Combine the ingredients in a dark glass bottle.

2. Shake when you want to use. Rinse with cool water.

3. After using the shampoo, use a natural conditioner followed by a vinegar hair rinse.

Caution: Do not use rosemary or peppermint essential oil if you have epilepsy or high blood pressure.

Dandruff Homemade Shampoo

Ingredients:

1/2 cup of liquid castile soap

1/2 teaspoon vegetable glycerin

5 drops tea tree essential oil

2 drops lavender essential oil

2 drops rosemary essential oil

Directions:

1. Combine the ingredients in a dark glass bottle.

2. Shake when you want to use. Rinse with cool water.

3. After using the shampoo, use a natural conditioner followed by a vinegar hair rinse.

Caution: Do not use rosemary essential oil if you have epilepsy or high blood pressure.

Blonde Hair Herbal Homemade Shampoo

Ingredients:

1/4 cup distilled water

1 tablespoon dried calendula blossoms

1 tablespoon chamomile flowers

1 tablespoon lemon peel

1/2 cup of liquid castile soap

1/2 teaspoon vegetable glycerin

5 drops grapefruit seed extract

Directions:

1. In a small pot, combine the distilled water with the herbs then bring to a boil.

2. Remove from heat and set aside for 30 minutes to an hour to steep.

3. Strain into a medium bowl, add the remaining ingredients then whisk together gently.

4. Lasts up to 4 weeks if refrigerated.

5. Rinse with cool water after use.

Red Hair Herbal Homemade Shampoo

Ingredients:

1/4 cup distilled water

1 tablespoon dried calendula blossoms

1 tablespoon hibiscus flowers

1 tablespoon cinnamon bark

1/2 cup of liquid castile soap

1/2 teaspoon vegetable glycerin

5 drops grapefruit seed extract

Directions:

1. In a small pot, combine the distilled water with the herbs then bring to a boil.

2. Remove from heat and set aside for 30 minutes to an hour to steep.

3. Strain into a medium bowl, add the remaining ingredients then whisk together gently.

4. Lasts up to 4 weeks if refrigerated.

5. Rinse with cool water after use.

Dark Hair Herbal Homemade Shampoo

Ingredients:

1/4 cup distilled water

1 tablespoon black tea

1 tablespoon dried rosemary

1 tablespoon cloves

1/2 cup of liquid castile soap

1/2 teaspoon vegetable glycerin

5 drops grapefruit seed extract

Directions:

1. In a small pot, combine the distilled water with the herbs then bring to a boil.

2. Remove from heat and set aside for 30 minutes to an hour to steep.

3. Strain into a medium bowl, add the remaining ingredients then whisk together gently.

4. Lasts up to 4 weeks if refrigerated.

5. Rinse with cool water after use.

Gray Hair Herbal Homemade Shampoo

Ingredients:

1/4 cup distilled water

1 tablespoon dried sage

1 tablespoon dried rosemary

1 tablespoon thyme

1/2 cup of liquid castile soap

1/2 teaspoon vegetable glycerin

5 drops grapefruit seed extract

Directions:

1. In a small pot, combine the distilled water with the herbs then bring to a boil.

2. Remove from heat and set aside for 30 minutes to an hour to steep.

3. Strain into a medium bowl, add the remaining ingredients then whisk together gently.

4. Lasts up to 4 weeks if refrigerated.

5. Rinse with cool water after use.

DIY Beer Hair Rinse

The nutrients in hops strengthens hair and make it shinier.

Ingredients:

1/4 cup beer

1/4 cup water

2 tablespoon of apple cider vinegar

Directions:

1. Mix together the ingredients in a bowl.

2. Condition your hair and rinse it properly.

3. Now use this mixture as a final rinse.

Repeat once a week.

HOMEMADE HERBAL HAIR CONDITIONER RECIPES

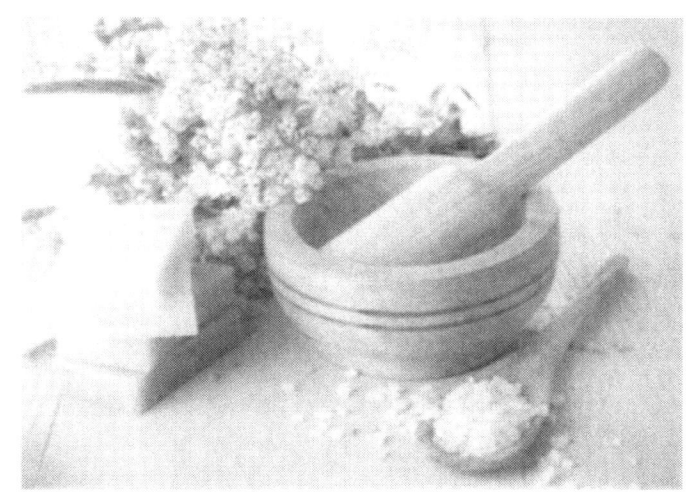

Natural Conditioners Customized For Your Hair

Making your own hair conditioners enables you to ensure that your hair is getting the right kind of treatment without using synthetic additives or unhealthy chemicals. These natural conditioners protect your hair from heat-styling, weather, poor diet, hormone fluctuations and so on. They also help to re-moisturizes dry hair, reduce breakage and split ends.

Lavender Coconut Conditioner

You only need a little bit of this conditioner and it is very moisturizing.

Ingredients:

1 cup of organic coconut oil

1 teaspoon of vitamin E oil

1 teaspoon of jojoba oil

5 drops of lavender essential oil

Directions:

1. In a mixing bowl, combine all the ingredients.

2. Mix on high for about 6-8 minutes.

3. Transfer to a jar and it is ready.

4. Refrigerate if you live in a warm area.

5. Usage: After shampooing and rinsing, apply a nickel-sized amount to your hair then work it in.

Simple Homemade Hair Conditioner

Makes about 8 ounces

Ingredients:

1 tablespoon apple cider vinegar

1 cup water

6-8 drops of essential oil (optional)

Directions:

1. Combine the ingredients in a bowl then transfer to a clean squirt bottle

2. Shake before you use.

3. Massage the conditioner into your hair and scalp for 1 or 2 minutes then rinse.

** You can add lovely fragrance to your DIY hair conditioner by using essential oils.

Oily/Greasy hair: Add 6-8 drops of lavender, bergamot, lemon, sandalwood, rosemary, ylang ylang or tea tree essential oil.

Dry hair/scalp: Add 6-8 drops of peppermint, tea tree, eucalyptus, sage, lemon or rosemary.

Herbal Infused Vinegar Hair Rinse

Ingredients:

3 or more tablespoons of dried herbs (see list below)

8 ounces apple cider vinegar

Directions:

1. In a glass jar, combine dried herbs and apple cider vinegar.

2. Cap tightly and let infuse for 2 weeks. Shake the jar every day.

3. Strain out the herbs after 2 weeks.

4. The infused vinegar can last for a year if stored in a cool and dry place.

5. Usage: Combine 1 tablespoon of herb-infused vinegar with 1 cup water. Massage it into your hair then rinse with water.

**Use 2-3 tablespoons of any combination of the herbs in the appropriate category:

Normal hair: Calendula, lavender, chamomile, sage, rosemary.

Dry hair/scalp: Chamomile, calendula, elder flowers, lavender, nettle, sage.

Oily hair/scalp: Chamomile, calendula, lemon balm, lemongrass, peppermint.

Quick Herb And Vinegar Hair Rinse

Ingredients:

2 tablespoons apple cider vinegar

2-3 tablespoons dried herbs of your choice**

2 cups of boiling water

Directions:

1. Add water to a saucepan and bring to a boil.

2. Remove from heat and add the vinegar and herbs

3. Cover and let steep for 30 minutes. Allow to cool before using.

4. Usage: Shampoo your hair then rinse it. Massage the hair rinse into your hair and scalp.

5. Rinse out with fresh water.

**Use 2-3 tablespoons of any combination of the herbs in the appropriate category:

Normal hair: Calendula, lavender, chamomile, sage, rosemary.

Dry hair/scalp: Chamomile, calendula, elder flowers, lavender, nettle, sage.

Oily hair/scalp: Chamomile, calendula, lemon balm, lemongrass, peppermint.

NATURAL HAIR LOSS RECIPES

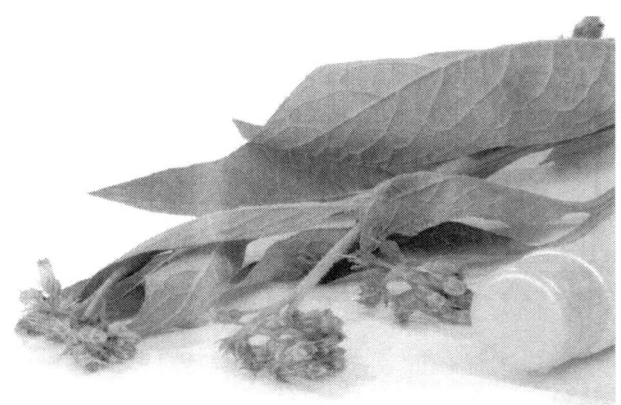

Have Fuller Hair Naturally

Harnessing the healing power of essential oils and herbs is vital if you want to slow down hair loss and have stronger and healthier hair. At the same time, you are also protecting your hair and scalp from harmful chemicals. Aromatherapy has been used successfully to treat alopecia areata and other hair problems. You can expect to have improved hair growth after a few months of using these recipes.

Coconut Scalp Treatment Oil

Coconut oil helps to prevent the loss of protein, which is a crucial factor in breaking and loss of hair.

Ingredients:

1 to 2 tablespoons virgin coconut oil

1 teaspoon lime juice

2 drops lemon essential oil

1 drop peppermint essential oil

Directions:

1. Put the coconut oil in a small glass bowl and warm it until it melts.

2. Stir in the other ingredients.

3. Massage it into your scalp and hair then leave it in for 30 minutes at least.

4. To retain more heat, cover your hair with a shower cap and then wrap it up with a wool cap.

Hibiscus Hair Pack

Ingredients

3 ounces hibiscus petal powder

6 teaspoons Aloe Vera gel

3 teaspoons honey

3 tablespoon plain yogurt

Coconut milk

10 drops rosemary essential oil

10 drops peppermint essential oil

10 drops lemon essential oil

Directions:

1. Combine the hibiscus petal powder, Aloe Vera gel, honey and plain yogurt in a small bowl.

2. Stir in enough coconut milk until you have a smooth paste then add the essential oils.

3. Massage the mixture into your hair. Leave it in for 30 minutes at least.

4. To retain more heat, cover your hair with a shower cap and then wrap it up with a wool cap.

5. Rinse your hair then shampoo to remove traces of the hair pack.

6. Do the treatment once a week.

Herbal Rinse For Hair Growth

Besides boosting hair growth, a herbal rinse is always beneficial regardless of your hair type. It balances the scalp's pH and reduces product build-up.

Ingredients:

2 cups distilled water

3 tablespoons dried sage

3 tablespoons dried rosemary

2 tablespoons apple cider vinegar

20 drops sage essential oil

20 drops rosemary essential oil

20 drops lavender essential oil

Directions:

1. In a small pot, combine the distilled water with the herbs then bring to a boil.

2. Remove from heat and set aside for 1-3 hours to steep.

3. Strain and pour the liquid into a dark glass bottle.

4. Add the apple cider vinegar and essential oils.

5. Shake the bottle very well to mix.

6. Usage: Shampoo and condition your hair then pour the herbal rinse your hair, using your fingers to gently rub it into your scalp. You can either rinse it or leave it in to dry.

Aloe Vera Scalp Massage Oil

Aloe Vera heals skin irritation, balances pH levels, cleanses the scalp and activates hair growth enzymes.

Ingredients:

1/4 cup Aloe Vera gel

1 teaspoon jojoba oil

3 drops cedarwood essential oil

10 drops rosemary essential oil

12 drops lavender essential oil

Directions:

1. Combine all the ingredients in a dark glass bottle.

2. Massage about 1 tablespoon into your scalp every night before bed.

3. Massage for about 10-15 minutes to stimulate blood flow and help the oil to penetrate deeply.

Lavender And Birch Nourishing Hair Lotion

Combine the wonderful benefits of lavender and birch in this lotion to prevent and cure dandruff, heal scalp irritations or infections, strengthen hair roots and promote hair growth.

Ingredients:

2 teaspoons of dried birch leaves

2 teaspoons of dried lavender blossoms

2 tablespoons of apple cider vinegar

A couple drops of lavender essential oil

Directions:

1. Combine the birch leaves and lavender blossoms in a clean glass bottle.

2. Pour the vinegar over the herbs, cover the lid tightly and place it in a cool and dry location away from direct sunlight.

3. After 1 week, strain the mixture to remove herbs then add a few drops of lavender essential oil.

4. When you want to use, add 1 part of the herbal mixture to 2 parts of water and massage it into your scalp. Do not rinse.

OTHER NATURAL HAIR CARE TREATMENT RECIPES

Organic Remedies For Your Hair

You can improve appearance, restore hair shine, relieve dandruff and slow down graying with the recipes in this section.

Hot Oil Conditioning Treatment

Ingredients:

2 tablespoons almond or jojoba oil

6 drops sandalwood essential oil

3 drops palmarosa essential oil

1 drop ylang ylang essential oil

Directions:

1. Combine the ingredients in a small glass cup.

2. Put the glass cup in a bowl of very hot water. Stir the mixture together as it becomes warm.

3. Usage: Apply to dry or damp hair and leave it on for at least 20 minutes.

4. To retain more heat, cover your hair with a shower cap and then wrap it up with a wool cap. If your hair is really dry, you can leave it

on for 2-3 hours or overnight. Place a towel on your pillow to protect it.

5. Wash it out with water and some shampoo.

Honey Conditioning Hair Pack

Ingredients:

1 tablespoon almond or jojoba oil

2 tablespoons honey

1 egg yolk

3 drops rosemary essential oil

3 drops lavender essential oil

Directions:

1. Beat together the oil, honey and egg yolk then stir in essential oils.

2. Usage: Dampen your hair then massage into your hair. Leave it on for at least 20 minutes.

3. To retain more heat, cover your hair with a shower cap and then wrap it up with a wool cap.

4. Wash it out with water and some shampoo.

Oily Hair Minty Hair Rinse

Ingredients:

2 cups distilled water

3 tablespoons dried peppermint

3 tablespoons rosemary

2 tablespoons apple cider vinegar

10 drops peppermint essential oil

5 drops tea tree essential oil

5 drops rosemary essential oil

Directions:

1. In a small pot, combine the distilled water with the herbs then bring to a boil.

2. Remove from heat and set aside for about 1 hour to steep.

3. Strain and pour the liquid into a dark glass bottle.

4. Add the apple cider vinegar and essential oils.

5. Shake the bottle very well to mix.

6. Usage: Shampoo and condition your hair then pour the herbal rinse your hair, using your fingers to gently rub it into your scalp. Rinse with water.

Dandruff Pre-Shampoo Treatment

Ingredients:

1 tablespoon of sesame oil

1 tablespoon of lemon juice

5 drops of ginger essential oil

Directions:

1. Combine everything in a small glass bottle and shake well.

2. Usage: Massage it into the scalp, leave it on to dry then shampoo.

3. Use the treatment 3-4 times every week.

Witch Hazel Dandruff Scalp Treatment

Ingredients:

1/2 cup witch hazel

20 drops tea tree essential oil

20 drops lavender essential oil

10 drops lemon essential oil

10 drops rosemary essential oil

Directions:

1. Combine all the ingredients in dark glass bottle.

2. Massage about 1 teaspoon into your scalp, just before bed.

3. Do this every night until the dandruff has cleared.

Homemade Nourishing Hair Treatment

Use this treatment weekly if you have dry hair. It softens and nourishes.

Ingredients:

2 tablespoons of olive oil (extra virgin)

1 tablespoon of coconut oil

Directions:

1. Add the olive oil to a small bowl.

2. Scoop the coconut oil in your palm and rub your hands together to warm it up.

3. Now put your hands in the olive oil to mix the two oils together.

4. Rub the mixture into your hair. Avoid the scalp and focus on the length and ends of the hair.

5. Comb through to distribute properly.

6. Cover your head with plastic wrap and leave the treatment on for at least 3-4 hours or overnight.

7. Shampoo and condition your hair.

Homemade Shealoe Butter For Hair

This body butter is good for your hair and skin. It moisturizes hair and skin, heals and soothes the skin, provides hold for hair styling and can be used as a sealer for hair.

Ingredients:

1/2 cup Shea butter

2 tablespoons coconut oil

1 teaspoon of honey (also helps to preserve)

1/4 cup of Aloe Vera juice

4 drops of tea tree essential oil (preservative for preventing mold)

Directions:

1. Create a double boiler by boiling water in a small pot and placing a glass bowl over it.

2. Add the Shea butter and coconut oil to the glass bowl so they can melt.

3. Add the honey and stir gently.

4. Remove the bowl from the heat then add Aloe Vera juice.

5. Mix well with a hand mixer. Let cool for about 30 minutes then add tea tree oil.

6. Scoop into an air tight container and refrigerate for a few hours before storing in a cool, dry place.

NATURAL HAIR DYE RECIPES

All-Natural Coloring For Your hair

Research has shown that chemical dyes can be harmful to your body over time. This is why it is important to know how to make your own natural hair dyes. Although, you won't get instant results with these recipes, repeated use will give you a shade that you will like.

Henna Hair Coloring

Henna is available for all hair colors. It provides the fasted way to dye hair naturally. It conditions deeply and gives the hair a rich shine.

Directions:

1. Buy henna hair coloring from trusted suppliers and follow the directions on the package.

Caution: Do not use for hair that is more than 10% gray. Do not use if you have already dyed your hair with commercial hair color.

Natural Remedy To Darken Gray Hair

This treatment can slow down or even reverse gray hair. Use it in conjunction with the Gray Hair Herbal Homemade Shampoo recipe and natural conditioner.

Ingredients:

2 cups of hot water

1/2 cup dried rosemary

1/2 cup dried sage

Directions:

1. In a small pot, combine the distilled water with the herbs then simmer for 30 minutes.

2. Remove from heat and set aside for several hours to steep.

3. Strain and use the liquid as hair colorant.

4. Pour the liquid on your hair and leave it in until dried.

5. Rinse with water and dry. Use twice a week until you get the desired shade then maintain the color by using once a month.

Blonde Hair Natural Hair Dye

For lightening, brightening and highlighting blonde and also light brown hair. It also works as a herbal rinse to remove product buildup, balance the scalp's pH and enhance hair shine and manageability.

Ingredients:

2 cups of hot water

3 tablespoons dried calendula petals

3 tablespoons chamomile flowers

3 tablespoons chopped lemon peel

2 tablespoons apple cider vinegar

Directions:

1. In a small pot, combine the distilled water with the herbs then bring to a boil.

2. Remove from heat and set aside for 1-3 hours to steep.

3. Strain and pour the liquid into a dark glass bottle. Add the apple cider vinegar.

4. Usage: After conditioning, pour the liquid over your hair and gently massage it into your scalp. Rinse .

5. Use twice a week until you get the desired shade then maintain the color by using once a month.

Natural Sun Streaking

Ingredients:

2 tablespoons chamomile tea

Juice of 1 lemon

Directions:

1. Mix together the two ingredients.

2. You need an inexpensive straw hat that has many holes in it.

3. Usage: Pull strands of your hair through the holes in the straw hat. Now apply the chamomile/lemon mixture to the exposed strands of hair.

4. Sit in the sun for up to 2 hours.(Remember to use sunscreen)

Golden Hair Natural Hair Dye

Use this if you want to add a rich golden tint to blonde hair.

Ingredients:

2 cups of hot water

1 large pinch of saffron threads

1 tablespoon lemon juice

Directions:

1. Boil 2 cups of distilled water.

2. Place the saffron threads in a large jug then pour the hot water over. Let it soak for about 10 to 15 minutes.

3. Strain and add the lemon juice to the liquid.

4. Usage: Bend your head over a basin to catch the liquid. Use the saffron liquid to rinse your hair about 15 or 20 times.

5. After the last rinse, wring out your hair then leave it for about 15 minutes before rinsing with water.

6. Use twice a week until you get the desired shade then maintain the color by using once a month.

Red Hair Natural Hair Dye

Use this to add red-gold highlights to red hair, light brown and also brown hair.

Ingredients:

2 1/2 cups of hot water

3 tablespoons dried calendula petals

1/4 cup red wine

Directions:

1. In a small pot, combine the distilled water with the herbs then simmer for 20 minutes.

2. Let cool then strain and add the red wine to the liquid.

3. Usage: Use after shampooing and conditioning. Bend your head over a basin to catch the liquid. Use the calendula liquid to rinse your hair several times.

4. After the last rinse, wring out your hair then leave it for about 15 minutes before rinsing with water.

5. Use twice a week until you get the desired shade then maintain the color by using once a month.

Dark Hair Natural Hair Dye

This recipe is good for bringing out rich brown tones in your dark hair.

Ingredients:

2 1/2 cups of hot water

1/3 cup walnut shells or black tea

Directions:

1. In a small pot, combine the distilled water with the herbs then simmer for 20 minutes.

2. Let cool then strain.

3. Usage: Use after shampooing and conditioning. Bend your head over a basin to catch the liquid. Use the calendula liquid to rinse your hair several times.

4. After the last rinse, wring out your hair then leave it for about 15 minutes before rinsing with water.

5. Use twice a week until you get the desired shade then maintain the color by using once a month.

CPSIA information can be obtained at www.ICGtesting.com
Printed in the USA
LVOW10s1522260415

436148LV00012B/570/P